Derouicha MATMOUR
Mohamed KADARI
Dalila MIRAOUI

Cardiovascular drugs

Derouicha MATMOUR
Mohamed KADARI
Dalila MIRAOUI

Cardiovascular drugs

Compendium of Therapeutic Chemistry Volume 1 : Tome 1

ScienciaScripts

Imprint

Cover image: www.ingimage.com

This book is a translation from the original published under ISBN 978-620-2-53226-6.

Publisher:
Sciencia Scripts
is a trademark of
Dodo Books Indian Ocean Ltd. and OmniScriptum S.R.L publishing group

120 High Road, East Finchley, London, N2 9ED, United Kingdom
Str. Armeneasca 28/1, office 1, Chisinau MD-2012, Republic of Moldova, Europe
Managing Directors: Ieva Konstantinova, Victoria Ursu
info@omniscriptum.com

Printed at: see last page
ISBN: 978-620-8-57779-7

Contents

Foreword

Therapeutic Chemistry is a key scientific discipline in the development of new medicines. Its aim is to discover new drugs or to improve the efficacy and safety of existing drugs by modifying their chemical structure. It is therefore a key area in the development of new treatments for a variety of diseases, such as cardiovascular diseases, cancer, neurological diseases, infections, etc.

This book, entitled *"Abrégé de Chimie Thérapeutique, Volume 1 : Tome 1 : Médicaments du Système Cardio- Vasculaire"*, is part a collection *of Abrégé de Chimie Thérapeutique* dealing with the different therapeutic classes of drugs.

This Volume 1: Tome 1 is therefore devoted specifically to the treatment of diseases of the *Cardiovascular System* such as arterial hypertension, namely diuretics, beta-blockers and central anti-hypertensives. Each chapter deals successively with a physio-pathological reminder, the history of discovery, pharmaco-chemical classification, the main molecules marketed, study of the leader, mechanism of action, study of the structure-activity relationship, etc.

indications, contraindications and side effects.

It is aimed primarily at students and residents in the medical sciences, particularly pharmacy and medicine.

Obviously, the authors are aware that this summary covers only part of the very broad field of drugs for the Cardiovascular System, which can be found in a more comprehensive manner in numerous treatises. We must also take into account the impressive development of research into new treatments for these diseases, with many promising advances.

While I hope that this book will be useful, students with clear and precise information on drugs for the *Cardiovascular System*, I would like to thank the authors for their deep commitment and their exceptional professionalism, which have made it possible to produce the first volume of *the Abrégé de Chimie Thérapeutique*, which will be followed by a second volume covering the rest of the therapeutic classes, such as anticoagulants, platelet anti-aggregants, fibrinolytics, etc., in the same volume.

Prof. DELLAOUI Yahia

Pharmacist Professor of Therapeutic Chemistry Faculty of Medicine, Oran

Foreword

The aim of *Therapeutic Chemistry* is to discover, develop and interpret the mode of action and the relationship between chemical structure and therapeutic activity of pharmacologically active molecules obtained by chemical synthesis or hemi-synthesis. On an industrial scale, *Therapeutic Chemistry* deals with the manufacture and quality control of raw materials for pharmaceutical use, including active ingredients and excipients.

This *Compendium of Therapeutic Chemistry* comprises several volumes covering the different therapeutic classes of drugs, the first of which is devoted to *Cardiovascular System Drugs.*

In each volume, *the Abrégé de Chimie Thérapeutique* describes the physio-pathology of the disease, the main drugs used, the main routes of chemical synthesis, the essential elements of quality control, the mechanism of action, the structure-activity relationship, the main indications, contraindications and undesirable effects.

The Compendium of Therapeutic Chemistry is intended for students of *Pharmacy, Medicine, Pharmaceutical Chemistry, Public Health Pharmacy Preparators* and post-graduate residents in Therapeutic Chemistry, Pharmacology, Cardiology, Nephrology and Internal Medicine, as well as drug professionals interested in the design, quality control and rational use of active ingredients.

Editorial Committee

The following people took part in the preparation and production of this book

Abrégé de Chimie Thérapeutique,

Volume 1

Medicines for the Cardiovascular System "

Dr. Derouicha MATMOUR
Dr. Mohamed KADARI
Dr. Dalila MIRAOUI
Prof. Houari TOUMI
Sidi Bel-Abbès Faculty of Medicine

Faculty of Medicine of Sidi

Bel-Abbès

Faculty of Medicine of Sidi

Bel-Abbès

Faculty of Medicine, Oran

Introduction to Volume 1 : Tome1

his first volume *of the Abrégé de Chimie Thérapeutique* is devoted to *drugs for the cardiovascular system*, which are of particular clinical importance in the long-term treatment of cardiovascular disease, one of the leading causes of mortality worldwide.

Three chapters are described in this Volume 1: Volume 1, drugs: diuretics, beta-blockers and central antihypertensives.

Each chapter deals successively with :

— General information on the therapeutic class and a physio-pathological reminder of the pathology concerned;

— History of discovery, pharmacochemical classification and main molecules marketed;

— Study of the leader for each class, i.e. its chemical synthesis and quality control according to the European Pharmacopoeia 9th edition;

— Molecular mechanism of action and study of the chemical structure-therapeutic activity relationship ;

- Main indications, contraindications, side effects and finally a conclusion and outlook.

An alphabetical index is included at the end of the book, making it easier to search and access information by INN or proprietary name.

List of Authors

The following people took part in the preparation and drafting of this report

Volume 1: Volume 1 entitled :

"Medicines for the Cardiovascular System

Dr. Derouicha MATMOUR
Dr. Mohamed KADARI
Dr. Dalila MIRAOUI
Prof. Houari TOUMI
Sidi Bel-Abbès Faculty of Medicine

Faculty of Medicine of Sidi

Bel-Abbès

Faculty of Medicine of Sidi

Bel-Abbès

Faculty of Medicine, Oran

Reading Committee

The following people took part in the reading of this book entitled :
"Abrégé de Chimie Thérapeutique, Volume1 : Tome 1
Medicines for the Cardiovascular System "

Prof. Karim MEGHACHOU
Sidi Bel-Abbès Faculty of Medicine

Prof. Ahmed OUGHILAS
Sidi Bel-Abbès Faculty of Medicine

Tribute

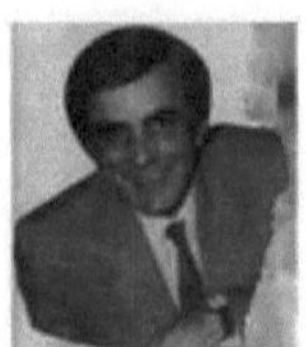

At the end of writing this book entitled *"Abrégé de Chimie Thérapeutique"*, I would like to pay tribute to *Professor Ali GHERIB*, the first *Professor of Therapeutic Chemistry* Algeria gained independence, who passed away on 12 February 1991 at the CHU Mustapha in Algiers.

Professor Ali Gherib obtained his state diploma in pharmacy in June 1964 from the Faculty of Medicine in Algiers. He took part in the training of all the classes of pharmacists trained from the time Algeria gained independence until the day he died, in his office at the Mustapha University Hospital in Algiers.

In 1967, *Prof. Ali Gherib* passed the competitive examination for the agrégation in Therapeutic Chemistry.

He was immediately appointed head pharmacist of the Central Biology Laboratory at the Mustapha University Hospital, which enabled him to rise to the rank of associate lecturer on November 1, 1967, and then trainee professor before being awarded tenure in November 1971. Since then, he has been one of the pillars of the Algerian pharmaceutical family, and a founder of the Société Algérienne de Pharmacie and the Fédération des Pharmaciens du Maghreb.

Dear Professor, please accept the expression of our sincere gratitude and testimony of respect for your career. We owe you and we will never forget you !!!

Peace to your soul !!!

Dr. Derouicha MATMOUR

Pharmacist Therapist who has never seen you !!!

Chapter 1

Diuretic drugs

1. Introduction

Diuretics are drugs used to treat redemas of various origins, and have become the mainstay of treatment for hypertension, despite successive advent of three new classes of antihypertensive drugs: β-blockers, angiotensin-converting enzyme inhibitors and calcium antagonists.

Before looking at the main diuretics, a reminder of the physiology of the nephron is necessary.

2. Anatomo-physiological reminder

2.1. Anatomy of the nephron

The nephron is the functional unit of the kidney, divided between the cortex and the medulla. The vascular part of the nephron consists of the glomerulus and the tubular part of the nephron consists of several segments ***(Figure 1)***:

- Bowman capsule ;
- Proximal contour tube (TCP) ;
- U-shaped *HENLÉ* handle (AH) in the medulla;
- Distal bypass tube (DBT) leading into the collecting duct (CD).

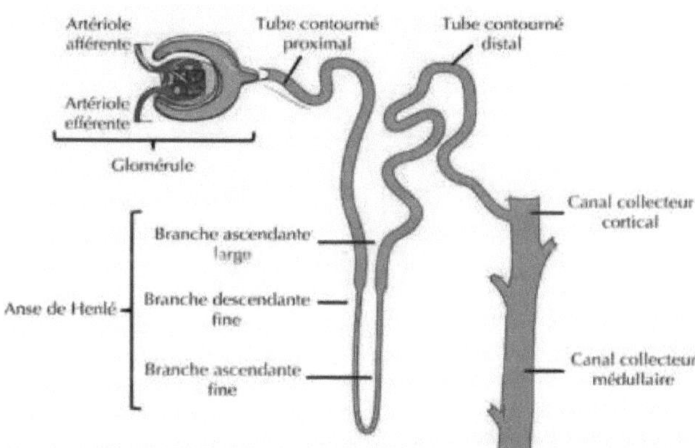

Figure 1: Different parts of the nephron (Servier Medical Art).

2.2. Functions of the nephron

Homeostasis of blood volume is an essential function of the nephron, which controls sodium and water excretion and thus ensures a state of balance between digestive intake and urinary elimination.

2.2.1. Glomerular filtration

The flow filtered by the glomeruli represents 1/5th of the renal plasma flow, i.e. approximately 120 $mL.min^{-1}$.

The osmolarity of the glomerular ultrafiltrate and its electrolyte concentration are identical to those of plasma: 180 litres/24 h

contains 600g of excreted NaCl, a high level that underlines the importance of the reabsorption function.

2.2.2. Tubular reabsorption and secretion

This passage mechanism occurs either passively by osmotic diffusion (water reabsorption), or by passive transport according to the electro-chemical gradient (Cl^- or urea), or by active transport requiring energy (glucose transport) ***(figure 2)***.

Reabsorption involves 99% of filtered water and 99.5% of filtered sodium. Most solutes are reabsorbed in the proximal convoluted tubule and in the loop of *HENLÉ*.

2.2.3. TCP: 65% water, 65% sodium and 65% potassium ;

2.2.4. Anse de *HENLÉ*: 15% water, 30% sodium and 25% potassium;

2.2.5. TCD and CC: final adjustment of the amount of sodium.

Segmental reabsorption of $Ca^{(2+)}$) and Mg^{2+} is comparable to that of sodium, but with slight differences. Tubular secretion occurs via transport systems for weak acids and bases such as urea, creatinine and uric acid ***(Figure 2)***.

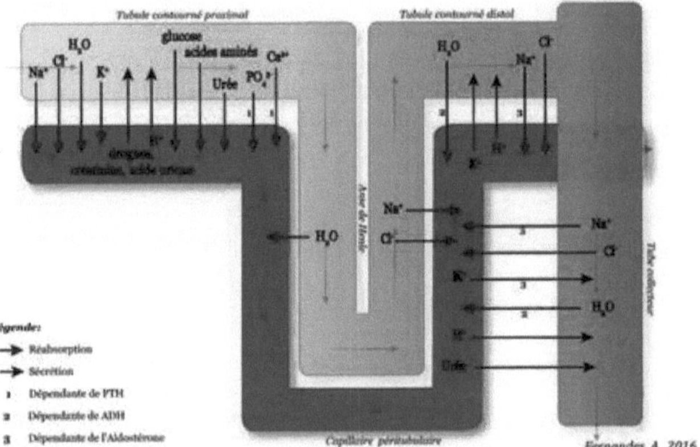

Figure 2. Main substances reabsorbed and secreted (Fernandes A, 2016).

2.3. Regulation mechanisms

2.3.1. Glomerulotubular balance

The balance that is established between the rate of filtration and tubular reabsorption maintains stable urinary excretion; this **"Glomerulotubular Balance"** ensures that for every decrease in the load filtered, there is a proportional decrease in the quantity reabsorbed.

2.3.2. Hormonal regulation

1. Renin-angiotensin-aldosterone system (RAAS)

Renin, secreted by the juxta-glomerular apparatus in response to variations in blood volume, activates circulating angiotensinogen of hepatic origin by proteolysis; the conversion enzyme converts the angiotensin I released into angiotensin II ***(Figure 3)***.

Angiotensin II exerts powerful vasoconstrictive effects (via its AT1 receptor) and stimulates adrenal cortical secretion of aldosterone, favouring retention of Na^+ and secretion of K^+ and H^+ . Stimuli for renin secretion are :

- Hypovolaemia or a drop in blood pressure;
- The sympathetic nervous system ;
- The increase in NaCl concentration in the macula densa (= tubulo-glomerular *feedback*).

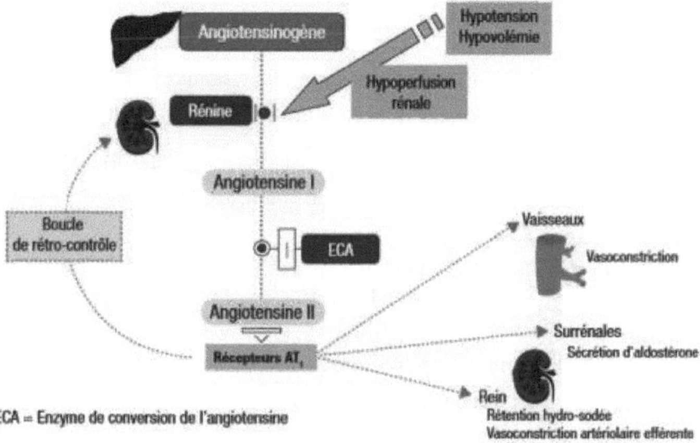

Figure 3. Physiology of the renin-angiotensin-aldosterone system (Collège Universitaire des Enseignants de Néphrologie, 2010).

2. Antidiuretic hormone (ADH): Arginine-vasopressin

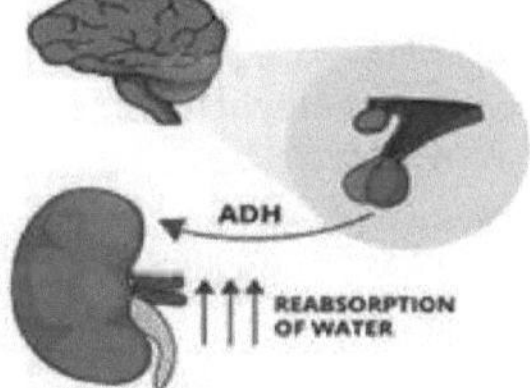

Figure 4. Physiology of antidiuretic hormone (iStock, 2018).

Antidiuretic hormone, or vasopressin, is a hormone produced by the hypothalamus and stored in the pituitary gland. It promotes water reabsorption by acting on the TCD ***(Figure 4)***.

3. Prostaglandins (PG)

The main effect of PGs is to modulate the action of certain hormones on renal haemodynamics or tubular transport. PGs are mainly produced by medullary collecting duct cells and interstitial cells, and to a lesser extent in the cortex by mesangial and glomerular arteriolar cells. Some are :

- Vasodilators and hypotensives (prostacyclin) ;
- Others have a vasoconstrictive effect (thromboxane).

4. Renal kinin-kallikrein system

Kinins are vasodilators and increase renal blood flow, but reduce renal resistance and do not affect glomerular filtration. The effects of kinins are potentiated by conversion enzyme inhibitors, which prevent their degradation.

5. Atrial natriuretic factors (ANF)

These peptides are secreted by the atria and have a rapid, massive and lasting diuretic and natriuretic effect.

3. Main groups of diuretics

3.1. Definition

Diuretics have in common the property of increasing the elimination of sodium and water by the kidney. They do this by inhibiting the renal reabsorption of sodium.

This ability of diuretics to negate the hydrosodium balance explains why they are used in the treatment of redematous states, arterial hypertension and heart failure.

3.2. Classification of diuretics

3.2.1. Depending on the site of action in the nephron

There are four classes of diuretics, distinguished by their site of action.

1. Proximal diuretics

These are carbonic anhydrase inhibitors *(Acetazolamide: DIAMOX®*) and osmotic substances *(Mannitol).* They are not used in the treatment of oedematous syndromes of renal origin, nor in the treatment of hypertension.

2. Loop diuretics

Furosemide (LASILIX®), Bumetanide (BURINEX®), Piretanide (EURELIX®); they inhibit sodium reabsorption in the ascending branch of the loop of *HENLÉ*.

3. Thiazide diuretics

These are derivatives of benzothiazide, and are therefore sulphonamides: *Hydrochlorothiazide (ESIDREX®), Chlortalidone (HYGROTON),®*

Indapamide (FLUDEX®). They inhibit sodium reabsorption in the proximal part of the distal tube, at the level of the dilution segment.

4. Distal diuretics" cortical collecting tube diuretics

These include *Amiloride (MODAMINE®*) and the anti-aldosterone drugs *Spironolactone (ALDACTONE®) and Eplerenone (INSPRA).®* They have

have the ability oppose Na /K^{++} exchange. They inhibit sodium reabsorption in the terminal part of the distal convoluted tubule and especially in the collecting tubule, and some are competitive inhibitors of aldosterone.

3.2.2. Depending on their effect on kalaemia

<ι **Hyperkalemic diuretics**: these include:
- Osmotic diuretics ;
- Carbonic anhydrase inhibitors ;
- Loop diuretics ;
- Thiazide diuretics.

€ **Hypokalemic diuretics**: these include :
- Anti-aldosterones ;
- Related anti-aldosterones.

3.3. General mode of action

3.3.1. Sodium transport mechanisms

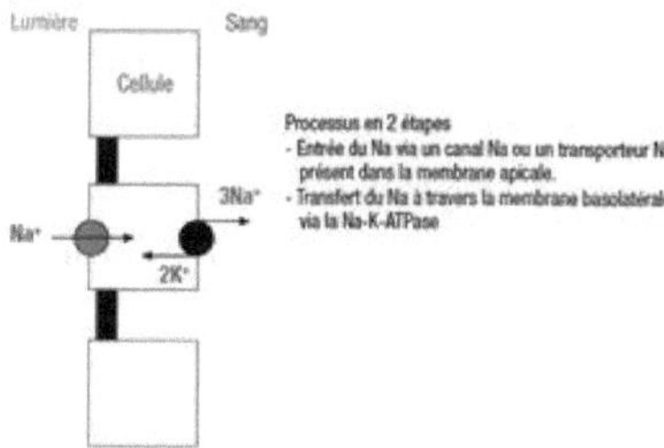

Figure 5. mechanisms of sodium reabsorption in the renal tubule (Collège Univer- sitaire des Enseignants de Néphrologie, 2018).

All sodium-transporting cells have Na-K-ATPase-dependent pumps on their basolateral membrane. These pumps are essential for sodium transport. Their functions are summarised ***in Figure 5***.

Each segment of the nephron has a unique sodium entry mechanism and the possibility of specifically inhibiting this step differentiates the different classes of diuretics ***(Figure 6).*** Most of the filtered Na is reabsorbed in the proximal convoluted tubule (60-65%) and the loop of *HENLÉ* (20%).

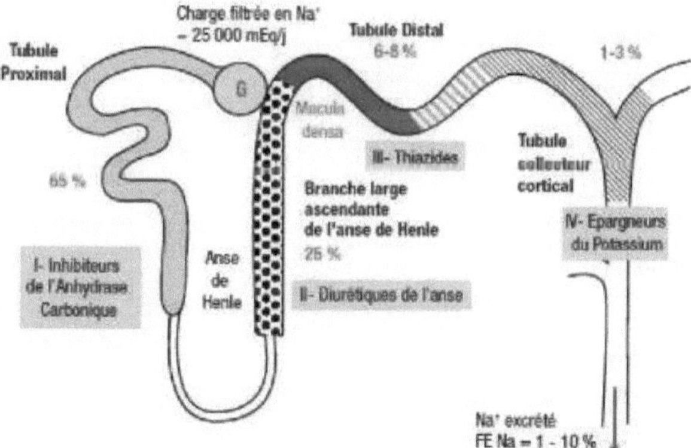

Figure 6. Site of action of diuretics (Collège Universitaire des Enseignants de Néphrologie, 2018).

3.3.2. Mechanism of action of diuretics

Diuretics reduce blood pressure essentially by reducing sodium reserves. Initially, they reduce pressure by reducing blood volume and cardiac output. After 6-8 weeks, cardiac output returns to normal and peripheral vascular resistance falls.

Sodium contributes to vascular resistance by increasing arteriolar vasoconstrictor tone and vascular reactivity under the action of endogenous vasoconstrictor substances such angiotensin II and catecholamines. This hyper-reactivity may be secondary to the calcium overload induced by chronic intracellular sodium overload. These effects are cancelled or reversed by diuretics or sodium restriction.

In patients with cardiac insufficiency, the kidney's capacity to eliminate sodium is impaired, resulting in fluid retention which leads to an increase in ventricular filling pressure, resulting an increase in cardiac work and a reduction in perfusion of the subendocardial layers, and exposing the heart to pulmonary oedema.

4. Carbonic anhydrase inhibitor diuretics

4.1. A reminder of carbonic anhydrase

Carbonic anhydrase is a zinc metalloprotein which catalyses the hydration of CO2 in the kidney, according to the following reaction in direction 1, it then controls the production of bicarbonates $HCO3^-$ and H ions$^+$ ***(figure 7)***.

Au niveau du rein →

$$CO_2 + H_2O \underset{2}{\overset{1}{\rightleftharpoons}} HO-C(=O)-OH \underset{2}{\overset{1}{\rightleftharpoons}} HO-C(=O)-O^- + H^+$$

Acide Carbonique — Bicarbonate

← Au niveau du poumon

Figure 7. CO2 hydration reaction under carbonic anhydrase.

It is present in the renal tubule, the ciliary body, the choroYd plexuses, the central nervous system and the digestive tract.

Inhibition of carbonic anhydrase favours the reaction in direction 2 and inhibitors have a diuretic effect when inhibition reaches 99% of the enzyme's activity, which reduces the concentration of $HCO3^-$ and H^+ ions. This inhibition leads to urinary elimination of bicarbonate and potassium, which are eliminated instead of protons (urine becomes highly alkaline). Urinary chloride elimination decreases at the expense of bicarbonate elimination. Urinary elimination of sodium increases moderately. Alkalinisation of the urine is accompanied by acidification of the plasma through loss of bicarbonates.

4.2. Story of discovery

Diuretic sulphonamides were developed when clinicians observed diuretic effects in patients treated with antibacterial sulphonamides (USA, 1938). In 1940, researchers proved that *sulphanilamide* acts as an inhibitor of carbonic anhydrase, which catalyses the reversible CO2 hydration reaction in the kidneys.

Carbonic anhydrase inhibitors are heterocyclic sulphonamides, characterised by a sulphonamide group carried by a heterocycle, usually nitrogenous and sulphurous. The derivatives of this group are most commonly used as antiglaucoma agents by reducing aqueous humour secretion.

Table I shows the main carbonic anhydrase inhibitors on the market. The leader in this series *Acetazolamide (DIAMOX®*) used systemically, while *Dorzolamide (TRUSOPT®*),

Dorzolamide + Timolol (COSOPT®) and *Brinzolamide (AZOPT®*) are used only as eye drops. In glaucoma, their efficacy is equivalent to that of β-blockers which act by a different mechanism.

Table I. Main marketed carbonic anhydrase inhibitors

Molecule DCI	Trade name and Pharmaceutical Form	Chemical Structure and Scientific Name
Acétazolamide **Chef de file**	**DIAMOX®** Comprimés à 250 mg Injectable à 100 mg/mL	*N*-(5-Sulfamoyl-1,3,4-thiadiazol-2-yl) acétamide.
Dorzolamide	**TRUSOPT®** Collyre à 20 mg/mL	7,7-dioxyde de (4*S*, 6*S*)- 4-(éthylamino)-6- méthyl-5,6-dihydro-4*H*-thiéno [2,3b] thiopyrane-2-sulfonamide.

Table I. Main carbonic anhydrase inhibitors on the market marketed (continued)

Molecule DCI	Trade name and Pharmaceutical Form	Chemical Structure and Scientific Name
Brinzolamide	**AZOPT®** Collyre à 10 mg/mL	(R)-4-(Éthylamino)-3,4- dihydro-2-(3-méthoxypropyl)-2H-thiéno [3,2-e]-1,2-thiazine-6-sulfonamide 1,1-dioxide.

4.3. Study of the lead partner

ACETAZOLAMIDE : DIAMOX®

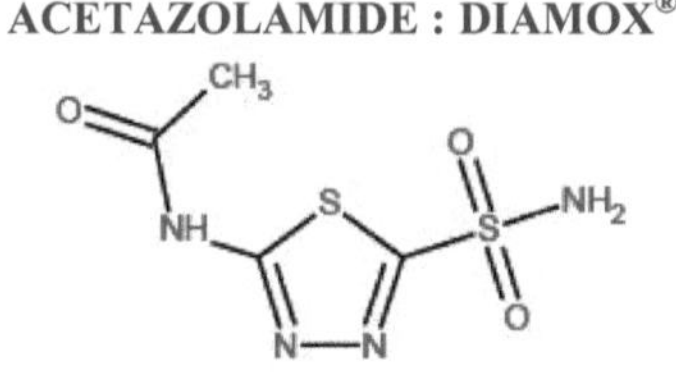

2-acetylamino-5-sulfamoyl-1,3,4-thiadiazole

Figure 8. Chemical structure of acetazolamide.

4.3.1. Chemical synthesis

Acetazolamide is synthesised in three main stages:

1. **Synthesis of intermediate 1:** ***2-Acetamido-5-mercaptothiadiazole***

The synthesis of intermediate 1 called "*2-Acetamido-5-mercapto-thiadiazole*" from thiosemicarbamide and carbon sulphide is illustrated *in* ***Figure 9.***

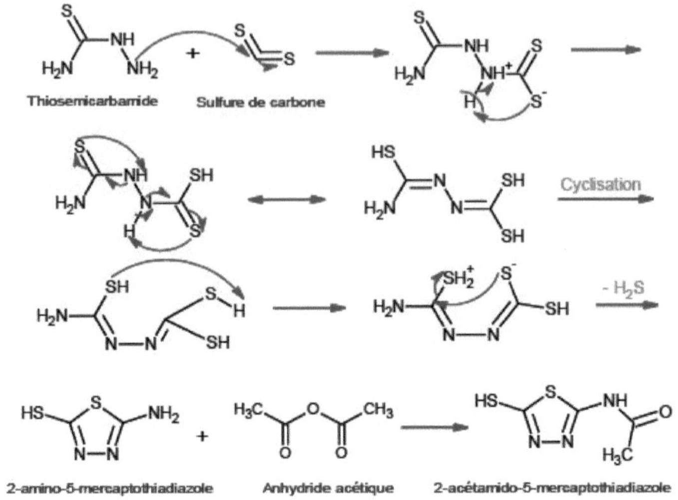

Figure 9. Synthesis of intermediate 1.

2. Intermediary 1

Intermediate 1 is treated with cold chlorine in an acetic medium to obtain the corresponding sulphochloride known as intermediate 2 ***(Figure 10).***

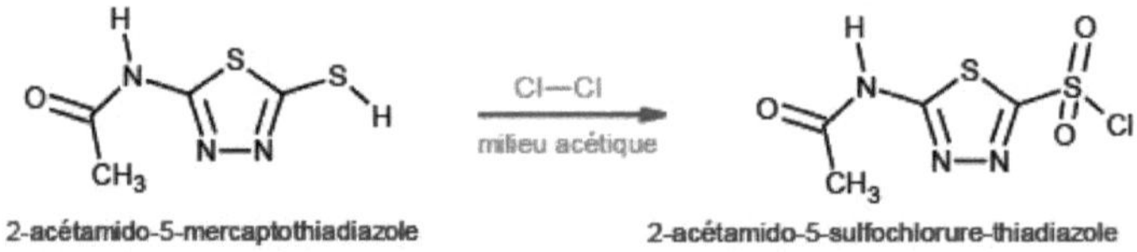

Figure 10. Chlorination of intermediate 1.

3. Action of cold ammonia

Treatment of intermediate 2 with cold ammonia produces *Acetazolamide* by a nucleophilic substitution reaction ***(Figure 11).***

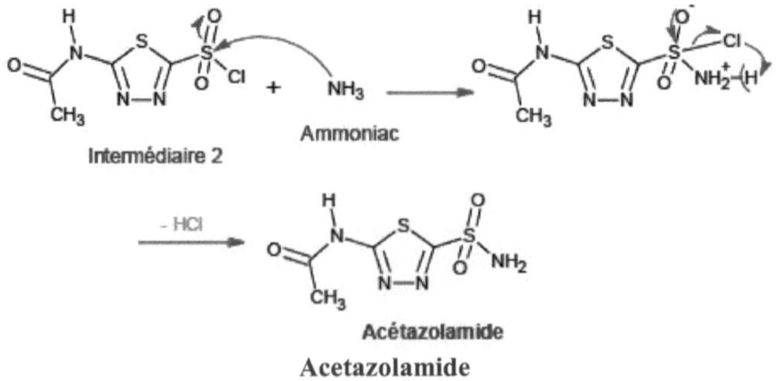

Acetazolamide

Figure 11. Action of ammonia to obtain acetazolamide.

4.3.2. Analytical control

1. **Physico-chemical properties**

Acetazolamide is a white crystalline powder, sparingly soluble in water and sparingly soluble in 96% ethanol. It dissolves in dilute alkali hydroxide solutions. *Acetazolamide* **is polymorphic**.

2. **Identification**

— Ultraviolet absorption maximum at 240 nm in 0.01 M NaOH solution.

— Infrared spectrophotometry by comparison with the spectrum of *Acetazolamide Chemical Reference Substance (CRS)*.

— Identification of the sulphonamide function: formation of a blue-green precipitate by adding 0.1 mL of dilute NaOH solution and 0.1 mL of CuSO4 solution.

3. **Test**

- Assay of related substances by liquid chromatography
- Test for sulphates, loss on drying and sulphuric ash.

4. **Dosage**

Titration by potentiometry with 0.1 M ethanolic sodium hydroxide solution.

4.3.3. Indications

Acetazolamide is used therapeutically in specific indications:

— Chronic glaucoma, because it reduces the secretion of aqueous humour;

- Cerebral oedema and mountain sickness, as it reduces the formation of cerebrospinal fluid in the choroYd plexuses and improves the pulmonary ventilation by lowering of plasma pH and increased sensitivity of chemoreceptors to hypoxia;

— Certain intractable epilepsies, possibly due to the conservation of Cl^- ions;

- Certain hypercapnia by promoting plasma acidification.

4.3.4. Contraindications

- Hypersensitivity *to acetazolamide* or sulphonamides
- Severe hepatic, renal or adrenal insufficiency
- History of renal colic
- First trimester of pregnancy.

4.3.5. Undesirable effects

Apart from the hydo-electrolytic risks, rare disturbances :

— Blood: thrombocytopenic purpura ;

— Cutaneous: necrotizing vasculitis ;

— Central: drowsiness, dizziness, agitation or depression;

— Digestive: diarrhoea ;

- Temporary myopia may occur.

5. Loop diuretics

5.1. Story of discovery

Loop diuretics are mainly represented by *Furosemide (LASILIX®*) and its relatives: *Bumetanide (BURINEX®*) and *Piretanide (EURÉLIX®* ***) (Table II)***. *Furosemide* was discovered as a result of work by W. SIEDEL et al on sulphamoylanthranilic acids in 1965. It subsequently emerged that isomeric 3-amino-benzoic acids had the same diuretic profile: work by P.W.FEIT et al in Denmark in 1971. In this series, replacing the chlorine in position 4 with a phenoxyl group increased activity and led to the use of *Bumetanide.* A structural analogue, *Piretanide,* resulting from the replacement of the butylamine in 3 by pyrrolidine, was proposed in 1976 by R. MUSCHAWECK of the Hoechst group. *Azosemide*, another loop diuretic invented in 1981, has the carboxyl function of *Furosemide* replaced by a tetrazole ring and the heterocycle linked to the amino function is a thiofene ***(Figure 12).***

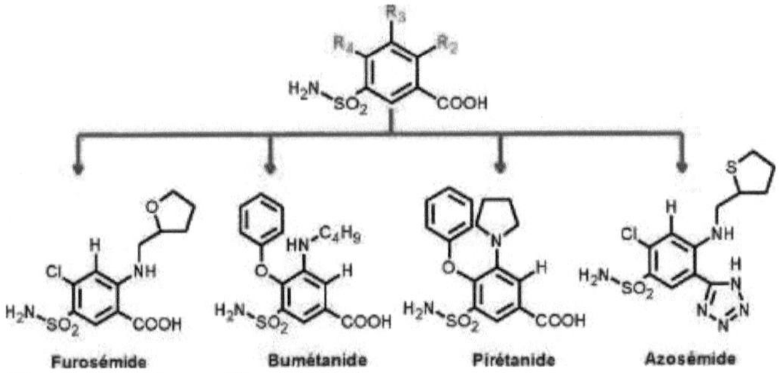

Furosémide Bumétanide Pirétanide Azosémide

Figure 12. Structural analogy of loop diuretics.

These are salidiuretic sulphonamides which act on the ascending branch of *the HENLÉ* loop, resulting in significant sodium excretion of up to 25-30% of the filtered sodium, which explains the name **"high ceiling diuretics"**.

They inhibit symport-type Na+/K+-2Cl⁻ co-transport by probably binding to the chloride site of the co-transporter. They reduce the reabsorption of sodium, potassium and chloride, increases urinary elimination. They also increase the urinary elimination of calcium and magnesium. Their action is rapid and of medium duration: 6-8 hours after oral administration. Because of the intensity and rapidity of their effects, they are indicated in the treatment of heart failure, particularly acute pulmonary oedema. Sustained-release preparations have less intense effects and a longer duration of action. They can be used to treat arterial hypertension. Their side effects are fairly similar to those of thiazide diuretics, but with a greater risk hyponatremia and dehydration.

Table II. Main loop diuretics.

Molecule DCI	Trade name and Pharmaceutical Form	Chemical Structure and Scientific Name
Furosémide Chef de file	**LASILIX®** Comprimés à 40 mg Gélules LP à 60 mg Injectable à 20 mg et 250 mg/mL	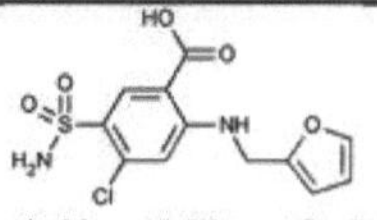 Acide 4-chloro-2-[(furan-2-ylméthyl) amino]-5-sulfamoylbenzoïque.
Bumétanide	**BURINEX®** Comprimés à 1 mg et 5mg Injectable à 2 mg/4mL	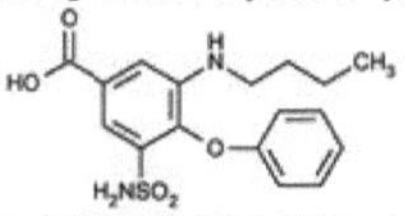 Acide 3-Butylamino-4-phénoxy-5-sulphamoyl-benzoïque.
Pirétanide	**EURÉLIX®** Gélules LP à 6 mg	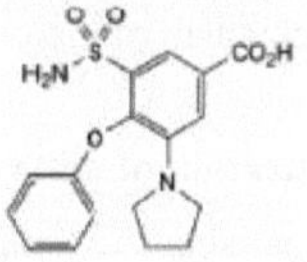 Acide 4-phénoxy-3-(pyrrolidin-1-yl)-5-sulfamoylbenzoïque.

5.2. Structure-activity relationship

- **Need for an acid group:** if the amine function is located at 2 (furfurylamine in *the* case of *Furosemide*), the carboxyl group can be replaced by a sulphonic group or tetrazole. On the other hand, if the amine is located in position 3 (butylamine in *the* case of *Bumetanide)*, carbon 1 must carry a carboxyl group.

- **Variability of the amine function:** unlike the amine function fixed at 2, the one fixed at 3 can vary (butylamine, pyrrolidine) without affecting the level of activity.

- **Nature of the substituents attached at 5 and 6:** this does not appear to be very decisive in the phamacomodulation of diuretic activity ***(Figure 12)***.

5.3. Mechanism of action

Entry of filtered NaCl into the cells of the ascending segment of the loop of *HENLÉ* is mediated by a Na-K-2Cl co-transporter located on the apical membrane of the cell. The energy for this transfer is provided by the favourable electrochemical sodium gradient (low intracellular concentration and electronegativity of the cell).

Loop diuretics directly inhibit the reabsorption of Na, K and Cl by competing with the Cl site of the co-transporter. In this way, they allow 20-25% of the filtered Na to be excreted.

They also have a significant effect on calcium and magnesium elimination (inhibition of NaCl reabsorption leads to inhibition of calcium and magnesium reabsorption). This action is very useful in the acute treatment of hypercalcaemia, unlike thiazides, which have the opposite effect, reducing urinary calcium excretion (***Figure 13).***

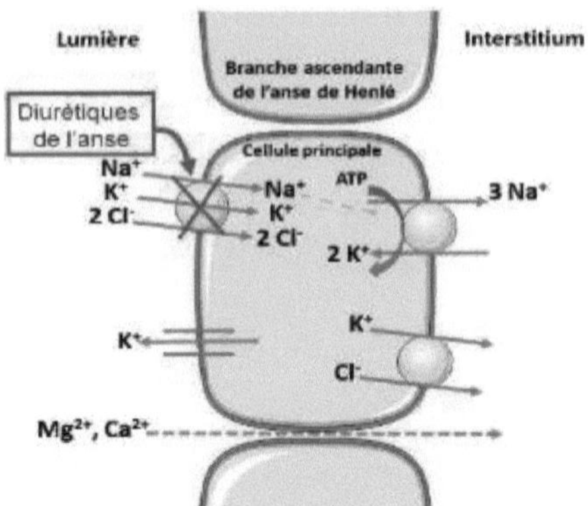

Figure 13. Mechanism of action of loop diuretics (Collège National de Pharmacologie Médicale, 2018).

Short onset and duration of action :

– IV route: takes about 5 minutes, maximum effect in 15 to 30 minutes, average elimination half-life of 1 hour and duration of effect of 3 hours;

– Per os: approximately 30 min delay, maximum effect in 1 h, average elimination half-life of 50 min and duration of effect of 7 h.

Their salidiuretic effect is proportional to the doses administered and persists in cases renal failure.

5.4. Study of the lead partner

FUROSEMIDE : LASILIX®

Acide 4-chloro-2-[(furan-2-ylméthyl)amino]-5-sulfamoylbenzoïque

4-Chloro-2-[(furan-2-ylmethyl)amino]-5-sulfamoylbenzoic acid

Figure 14. Chemical structure of Furosemide.

5.4.1. Chemical synthesis

Furosemide is synthesised in three main stages:

1. **Synthesis of intermediate 1**

The synthesis of intermediate 1 called *"2,4-dichloro-5-sulpho-chlorobenzoic acid"* by the action of sulphuric chlorohydrin on 2,4- dichlorobenzoic acid is illustrated *in* ***Figure 15***.

Acide 2,4-dichlorobenzoïque   Chlorhydrine sulfurique   Intermédiaire 1

Figure 15. Synthesis of intermediate 1.

2. **Treatment of intermediate 1 with ammonia**

Intermediate 1 is treated with cold ammonia produce intermediate 2 by a nucleophilic substitution reaction ***(Figure 16)***.

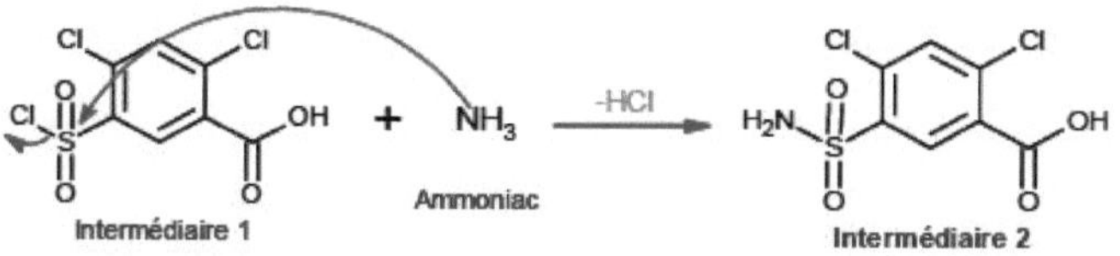

Figure 16. Synthesis of intermediate 2.

3. **Condensation of intermediate 2 with aminomethyl furan**

Condensation of intermediate 2 with aminomethyl furan produces *Furosemide* ***(Figure 17)***.

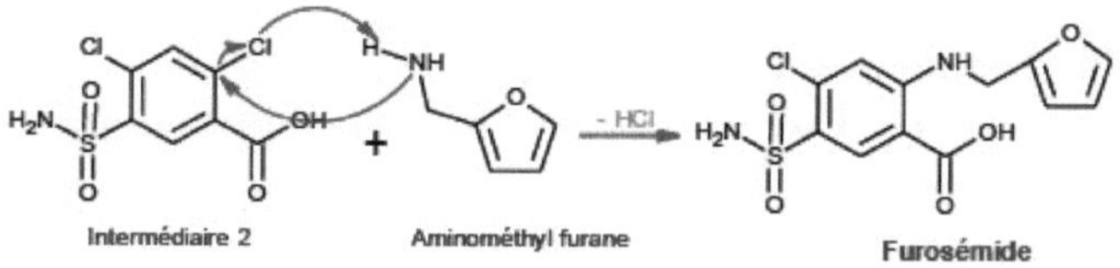

Figure 17. Production of Furosemide.

5.4.2. Analytical control

1. **Physico-chemical properties**

Furosemide is a white crystalline powder, insoluble in water, soluble in acetone, fairly soluble in 96% ethanol and practically insoluble in methylene chloride. It dissolves in dilute solutions of alkali hydroxides.

Furosemide **is polymorphic.**

2. **Identification**

— Ultraviolet absorption maxima at 228 nm, 270 nm and 333 nm in 4 g/L NaOH solution.

— Infrared spectrophotometry compared with the spectrum *of Furosemide SCR.*

— *Furosemide* develops a red-violet coloration on addition hot dilute HCl, 1 M NaOH and 1 mL 5 g/L sodium nitrite. After standing, 2 mL 25 g/L sulphamic acid and 1 mL 5 g/L naphthylethylenediamine dihydrochloride are added.

3. **Test**

- Assay of related substances by liquid chromatography
- Test for chlorides, sulphates, loss on drying and sulphuric ash.

4. **Dosage**

Titration by potentiometry with a 0.1M sodium hydroxide solution.

5.4.3. Indications

- Edema of cardiac or renal origin
- Edema of hepatic origin, most often in association with a potassium-sparing diuretic
- Hypercalcaemia.
- Arterial hypertension in patients with chronic renal failure, if contraindicated by diuretics

thiazides (creatinine less than 30 ml/min)

5.4.4. Contraindications

- Hypersensitivity to sulphonamides
- Acute functional renal failure
- Hepatic encephalopathy
- Hypovolaemia
- Dehydration
- Severe hypokalaemia and hyponatraemia.

5.4.5. Undesirable effects

- Decrease in kalaemia, possibly associated with cramps
- Dehydration may occur in the elderly
- Increase in blood glucose or 'uricemia
- Orthostatic hypotension
- At high doses: drop in blood levels of sodium (hyponatremia) and risk of behavioural problems
- Rarely: skin rash, photosensitisation and abnormal blood count.

5.4.6. Properties of Furosemide

Furosemide can be distinguished from other diuretics by :

- Rapid onset of action: diuresis is maximal one hour after ingestion and half an hour after injection of the product;
- Very high diuresis (x10) ;
- A small increase in dose leads to a significant increase in diuresis;
- Route of administration : oral, intramuscular and intravenous.

6. Thiazide diuretics

6.1. Story of discovery

Thiazide diuretics are mainly represented by *Hydrochlorothiazide (ESIDREX®*), the most widely prescribed and used, and its relatives: *Indapamide (FLUDEX®) and Ciclétanine (TENSTATEN®)* ***(Table III).*** Chlorothiazide is the prototype of the thiazides and was discovered by F.C. Novello and J.M. Sprague in 1957 during a systematic study of carbonic anhydrase inhibiting sulphonamides. It is characterised in particular by the presence of a halogen at 6 and a sulphonamide group at 7. The structural modifications carried out on the head of the series mainly concerned saturation of the 3,4 double bond by access to 3,4-dihydrobenzothiadiazines, mainly *Hydrochlorothiazide*, the most widely used therapeutically ***(figure 18).***

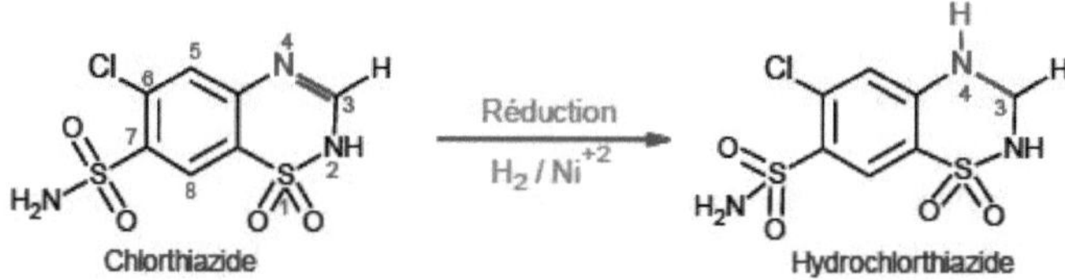

Figure 18. Saturation of chlorothiazide to produce hydrochlorothiazide.

Thiazide diuretics act at the level of the dilution segment (proximal segment of the TCD), by inhibiting the Cl^-/Na symport cotransport$^+$. They increase diuresis (less potent than loop diuretics), sodium excretion (natriuretics) and potassium excretion (kaliuretics). As a result, they induce contraction of extra-cellular volumes, which can lead to extra-cellular dehydration, functional renal failure and orthostatic arterial hypotension. They increase the risk hypokalaemia and hyponatraemia. They increase urinary elimination of magnesium but reduce that of calcium, which reduces the risk of fractures in the elderly.

Their diuretic effect is less rapid, less powerful, more gradual and more prolonged than loop diuretics, and their maximum effect is limited whatever the dose. Their main indication essential hypertension with preserved renal function. They are inactive in patients with renal failure.

Indapamide and *Ciclétanine* have little diuretic activity but a definite vasodilatory effect. They are indicated only in the treatment of , where their direct effect on vascular smooth fibres outweighs their diuretic effect.

Their adverse effects include hypokalaemia, hyperuricaemia, hypomagnesaemia, hyperglycaemia, hypercholesterolaemia, worsening of renal failure and the possibility of hyponatraemia in the elderly. Skin rashes and leukopenia have been reported in exceptional cases.

Table III. Main thiazide diuretics.

Molecule DCI	Trade name and Pharmaceutical Form	Chemical Structure and Scientific Name
Hydrochlorothiazide **Chef de file**	**ESIDREX®** Comprimés à 25 mg	6-Chloro-3,4-dihydro-2H-1,2,4 benzothiadiazine -7-sulfonamide 1,1-dioxide.
Indapamide	**FLUDEX®** Comprimés à 2 mg et 5 mg	4-Chloro-N-(2-méthyl-1-indolinyl)-3-sulfamoyl benzamide.
Ciclétanine	**TENSTATEN®** Gélules à 50 mg	1,3-dihydro-6-méthyl-7-hydroxy-3(4-chlorophényl) furo (3,4-d) pyridine.

6.2. Mechanism of action

In the distal tubule, entry of filtered sodium into the cell is mediated by a NaCl cotransporter located on the apical membrane.

Thiazide diuretics directly inhibit NaCl reabsorption through competition with the Cl site of the co-transporter. They indirectly stimulate calcium reabsorption (increase in proximal tubular reabsorption parallel to that of Na). Their effect is weak; they allow 5 to 10% of filtered sodium to be excreted.

Their diuretic effect and dose-response relationship are less significant than for loop diuretics. Their onset and duration of action are longer than for loop diuretics, and they are ineffective in cases renal failure ***(Figure 19).***

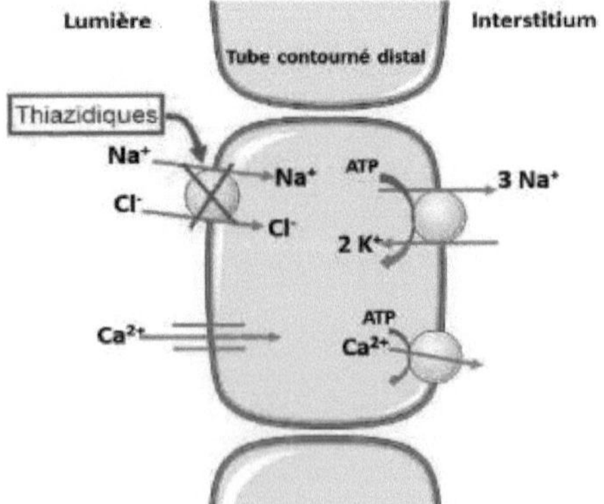

Figure 19. Mechanism of action of thiazide diuretics (Collège National de Pharmacologie Médicale, 2018).

6.3. Study of the lead partner

HYDROCHLORTHIAZIDE : ESIDREX®

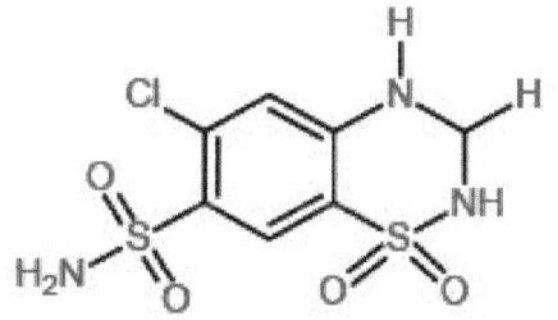

6-Chloro-3,4-dihydro-1,2,4-benzothiadiazine-7-sulfonamide-1,1-dioxi

6-Chloro-3,4-dihydro-1,2,4-benzothiadiazine-7-sulfonamide-1,1-dioxi

Figure 20. Chemical structure of Hydrochlorothiazide.

20.3.1. Chemical synthesis

Hydrochlorothiazide is synthesised by the action of formic acid on Salamide (Aminochlorobenzene-disulphonamide), intermediate 1 obtained is dehydrated to give *Chlorthiazide* which undergoes catalytic hydrogenation ***(figure 21)***.

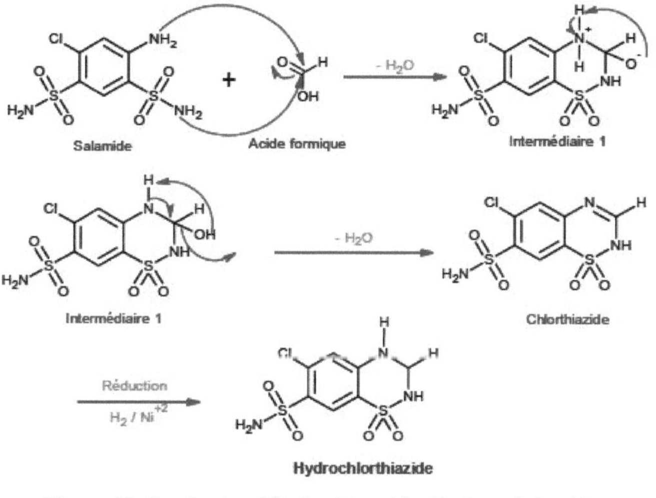

Salamide

Acide formique

- H_2O

Intermédiaire 1

Intermédiaire 1

- H_2O

Chlorthiazide

Réduction

H_2 / Ni^{+2}

Hydrochlorthiazide

Figure 21. Synthesis of Hydrochlorothiazide from Salamide.

6.3.2. Analytical control

1. Physico-chemical properties

Hydrochlorothiazide is a white crystalline powder, very slightly soluble in water, soluble in acetone and fairly soluble in 96% ethanol. It dissolves in dilute solutions of alkali hydroxides. *Hydrochlorothiazide* **is polymorphic.**

2. Identification

- Ultraviolet absorption maxima at 273 nm and 323 nm in 0.1 M NaOH solution.

- Infrared spectrophotometry compared with the spectrum of Hydrochlorothiazide SCR.

- Thin layer chromatography by dissolution in acetone and comparison with the control containing Hydrochlorothiazide SCR.

- Hydrochlorothiazide develops a violet colour when 0.5 g/L chromotropic acid sodium is added to a cooled mixture of 35 volumes of water and 65 volumes of sulphuric acid.

3. **Test**

- HPLC assay of related substances
- Test for acidity or alkalinity, chlorides, loss on drying and sulphuric ash.

4. **Dosage**

By liquid chromatography as indicated in the test for related substances.

6.3.3. Indications

- Edema of cardiac or renal origin.
- Edema of hepatic origin, most often in association with a potassium-sparing diuretic.
- High blood pressure.

6.3.4. Contraindications

- Hypersensitivity to sulphonamides
- Severe renal insufficiency
- Gestational oedema
- Pregnancy-induced hypertension
- Hypersensitivity or intolerance to gluten
- Hepatic encephalopathy.

7. Potassium-sparing diuretics

7.1. General

Potassium-sparing diuretics belong to two chemical series:

- Steroid diuretics are aldosterone antagonists known as antialdosterones: *Spironolactone (ALDACTONE)*® and *Canrenate of potassium canrenate (SOLUDACTONE);*®

- Non-steroidal diuretics or physiological aldosterone antagonists whose site of action is independent of aldosterone: *Amiloride (MODAMINE*®) and *Triamterene (CYCLOTERIAM*® *)* ***(Table IV).***

They are called distal diuretics because they act on the distal part of the nephron. They increase the urinary elimination of sodium and reduce that of potassium.

Because of their chemical structure, which is similar to that of steroid hormones, antialdosterones can cause endocrine side-effects, such as impotence and gynaecomastia in men, and menstrual disorders and amenorrhoea in women. They are indicated in the treatment of primary hyperaldosteronism or hyperaldosteronism secondary to cirrhosis, nephrotic syndrome or heart failure, as well as in the treatment of essential arterial hypertension.

Related antialdosterone drugs (*Amiloride* and *Triamterene)* are hyperkalaemic diuretics that can be used in combination with a hypokalaemic thiazide diuretic to reduce the risk of hypokalaemia. They also reduce urinary calcium losses.

Table IV. Main distal diuretics.

Molecule DCI	Trade name and Pharmaceutical Form	Chemical Structure and Scientific Name
Spironolactone	**ALDACTONE®** Comprimés à 50 mg et 75 mg	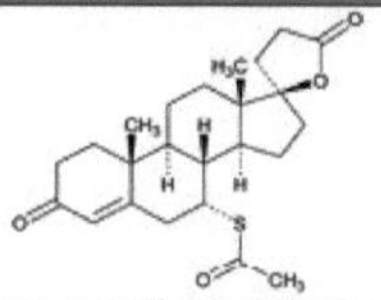 (2'R)-(Acétylsulfanyl)-3',4'-dihydro -5'H-spiro[androst-4-ène-17,2'-furane] -3,5'-dione.
Canrénoate de potassium	**SOLUDACTON®** Injectable à 50 mg/mL	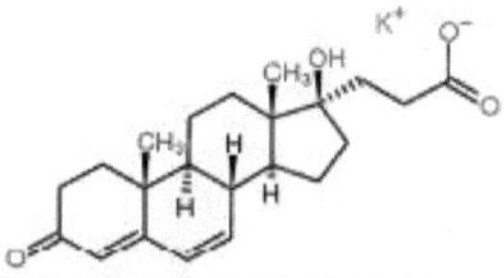 3-[(14-hydroxy-2,15-diméthyl-5-oxo-tétracyclo] heptadéca-6,8-dièn-14-yl] propanoate de potassium.
Amiloride	**MODAMIDE®** Comprimés à 5 mg	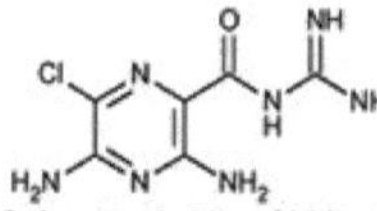 3,5-diamino-6-chloro-N-(diamino-méthylidène) pyrazine-2-carboxamide.
Triamtérène	**CYCLOTERIA®** Comprimés à 150 mg	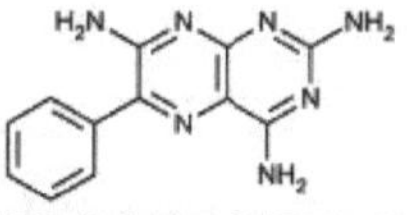 6-Phénylptéridine-2,4,7-triamine

7.2. Mechanism of action

They act at the level of the main cell in the cortical collecting tube. Entry of filtered sodium into these cells is mediated by the presence of an epithelial sodium channel (ENaC) on the apical membrane. Energy is supplied by the favourable Na gradient. The reabsorbed Na is then excreted from the cell by an Na-K- ATPase-dependent pump on the basolateral membrane. Aldosterone increases the number of sodium channels and Na-K-ATPase-dependent pumps.

- Physiological aldosterone antagonists (*Amiloride* and *Triamterene)* directly block the epithelial sodium channel.

- Antialdosterones (*Spironolactone* and *potassium*) oppose the action of aldosterone by competing with the intracytosolic mineralocorticoid receptor.

The natriuretic effect of these substances is weak, resulting in excretion of 1 to 3% of filtered sodium. They are mainly used in combination with thiazides to prevent urinary potassium leakage ***(Figure 22).***

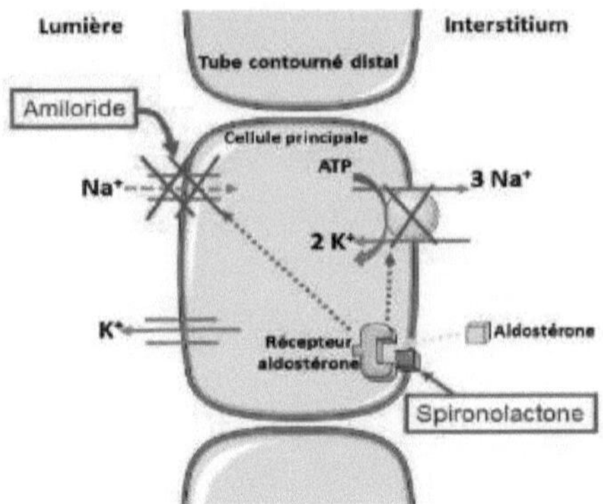

Figure 22. Mechanism of action of potassium-sparing diuretics (Collège National de Pharmacologie Médicale, 2018).

7.3. Study of the lead partner

AMILORIDE : MODAMIDE®

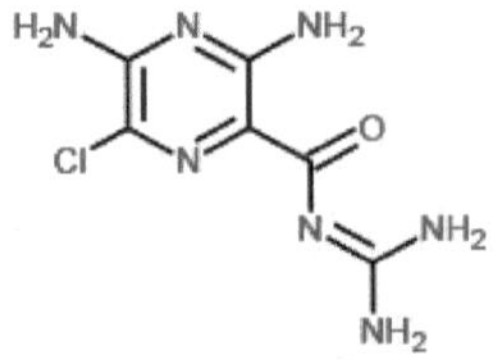

3,5-diamino-6-chloro-N-(diaminométhylidène) pyrazine-2-carboxamide

3,5-diamino-6-chloro-N-(diaminomethylidene) pyrazine-2-carboxamide

Figure 23. Chemical structure of Amiloride.

7.3.1. Chemical synthesis

Intermediate 1 is the key intermediate formed by 3-amino-5,6-dichloropyrazine-2-ethylcarboxylate. Aminolysis leads to the displacement of the chlorine activated by the carboxylate group in para giving intermediate 2 which is converted to *Amiloride* by heating in the presence of guanidine hydrochloride ***(figure 24)***.

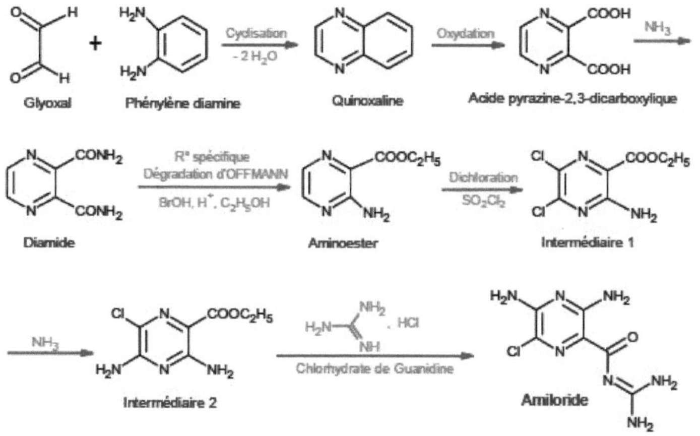

Figure 24. Amiloride synthesis.

7.3.2. Analytical control

1. Physico-chemical properties

Amiloride is a pale yellow or yellow-green powder, sparingly soluble in water and anhydrous ethanol, and practically insoluble in heptane.

2. Identification

- Infrared spectrophotometry compared with the spectrum *of SCR Amiloride.*

- Thin layer chromatography by dissolution in methanol and comparison with the control containing *Amiloride SCR.*

- *Amiloride* develops a yellow-green colouration on addition of 10 mL of a 200 g/L cetrimide solution, 0.25 mL dilute NaOH and 1 mL bromine water. The addition of 2 mL dilute HCl causes a dark yellow colour change and the solution fluoresces blue in ultraviolet light at 365 nm.

3. Test

- Testing of related substances by liquid chromatography - Testing for free acid, chlorides, water content and sulphuric ash.

4. Dosage

Titration by potentiometry with 0.1 M sodium hydroxide solution.

7.3.3. Indications

- Cardiac oedema
- Ascites and oedema in cirrhotics
- Hypertension
- Adjuvant to prevent potassium depletion in patients receiving thiazides or other antihypertensive diuretics for prolonged treatment.

7.3.4. Contraindications

- Hypersensitivity to *Amiloride*

- Hyperkalaemia greater than 5.5 mmol/L
- Severe renal insufficiency
- Congenital galactosemia
- Glucose or galactose malabsorption syndrome
- Lactase deficiency.

8. Conclusion

Diuretics are pharmacological agents designed to increase renal excretion of sodium and, consequently, water. There are three classes of diuretics: *loop diuretics, thiazide diuretics* and *potassium-sparing diuretics*. The criteria for choosing a diuretic are based on :

J **Action on kalaemia**

J **Timeframe and duration of action**

- Fast-acting (1 h) and short-acting (6 h): *Furosemide*
- Less rapid onset of action (3-12 h): *Amiloride*
- Delayed (3 days) but prolonged action: *Spironolactone*

L **The power to act**

- Powerful action even in cases of renal failure: Furosemide
- Moderate action, ineffective in cases of renal insufficiency: Thiazides
- Weakly natriuretic action but hyperkalaemic in cases of renal failure: related anti-aldosterones.

L **The risk accidents**

- These depend on the type of diuretic: hypokalaemia and hyperkalaemia.
- Those which depend on the potency of the action: hyponatremia, dehydration, hyperuricaemia, etc.

9. References

1. LE BEAUT G. Les Diurétiques. **In**: BRION JD, BUXERAUD J, CASTEL J et al. *Médicaments du Système Cardio-Vasculaire*, Paris: Tec & Doc, 1992, p. 3-104. (Traité de Chimie Thérapeutique, Volume 3).
2. KIRKIACHARIAN, Serge. Medicines for the Cardiovascular System. **In**: *Guide de Chimie Médicinale et Médicaments*, Paris: Tec & Doc, 2010, p. 269-279.
3. KIRKIACHARIAN, Serge and PIERI, François. Diuretics. **In**: *Pharmacologie et Thérapeutique.* 2th ed. Paris: Ellipses, 1992, p. 211224.
4. TAOUFIK, Jamal. Médicaments du Système Cardio-Vasculaire. **In**: *Précis de Chimie Thérapeutique*, Rabat: MEDIKA, 2007, p. 245-256.
5. MOULIN Bruno and PERALDI Marie-Noêlle. Elements of renal physiology. **In** : *Néphrologie.* 8ème éd **[On line].** Paris : Ellipses, 2018, p. 09-19. Available on : < http://cuen.fr/manuel/IMG/pdf/01 -nephro logie8e-editionchap1.pdf> (Accessed 11/12/2019).
6. MOULIN Bruno and PERALDI Marie-Noêlle. Diuretics. **In** : *Néphrologie.* 8ème éd **[En**

ligne]. Paris : Ellipses, 2018, p. 61-69. Available at:< http://cuen.fr/manuel/IMG/pdf/04-nephrologie-8e- editionchap4.pd> (Accessed 11/12/2019).

7. Collège des Enseignants de Cardiologie et Maladies Vasculaires. Item 176 : Prescription and monitoring of diuretics. [On line]. Université Médicale Virtuelle Francophone, Support de cours, 20112012, 10 p. Available at:< http://campus.cerimes.fr/cardiologieet etmaladiesvasculaires/enseignement/cardio176/site/htm l/cours.pdf> (Accessed 13/12/2019).

8. LECHAT, Philippe. *Pharmacologie.* *[***On-line].** Paris: Université Pierre et Marie Curie, Service de pharmacologie, Niveau DCEM1, 2006, 349 p. Available on : < http://www.chups.jussieu.fr/polys/pharmaco/ poly/Pharmaco.pdf> (Accessed 10/12/2019).

9. European Directorate for the Quality of Medicines and Healthcare. Acetazolamide monograph. **In**: *European Pharmacopoeia.* 9th ed. France: EDQM, 2018, p. 1751-1752.

10. European Directorate for the Quality of Medicines and Healthcare. Furosemide Product Monograph. **In**: *European Pharmacopoeia.* 9th ed. France: EDQM, 2018, p. 2768-2770.

11. European Directorate for the Quality of Medicines and Healthcare. Hydrochlorthiazide Product Monograph. **In** : *Pharmacopoeia*
9th ed. France: EDQM, 2018, p. 2888-2890.

12. European Directorate for the Quality of Medicines and Healthcare. Amiloride monograph. **In**: *European Pharmacopoeia.* 9th ed. France: EDQM, 2018, p. 1840-1842.

Chapter 2

Beta-Blocker drugs

1. Introduction

Beta-blockers are competitive but reversible inhibitors of the effects of catecholamines on beta-adrenergic receptors. This inhibition is attributable to a chemical relationship with adrenaline and noradrenaline, and consists of a specific blockade of the receptors for these amines.

The aim of treatment with beta-blockers is to protect the heart and the entire vascular nervous system from catecholamine discharges associated with stress or physical effort. Arterial hypertension and coronary insufficiency are the main indications.

2. Physiological reminder

Beta-adrenergic receptors β1 and β2 are seven-pass transmembrane receptors coupled to adenyl cyclase by a G protein. Stimulation of these receptors induces the formation of cyclic AMP from ATP, a second messenger that activates protein kinase A, which phosphorylates various proteins, accounting for the diversity of effects.

β1 receptors are preferential in the heart, kidneys and adipose tissue, while β2 receptors are predominant in the vascular and bronchial ***systems (Figure 1).***

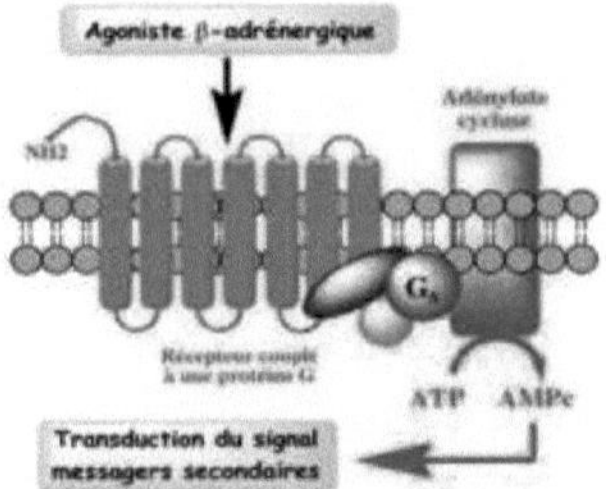

Figure 1: β-adrenergic receptor *(E. Jaspard, 2011).*

To understand the consequences of inhibiting β-receptors, we need to know the effects of stimulating them.

1. Stimulation of post-synaptic β_1 receptors leads to ***(Figure 2)***:

— Positive cardiac inotropic, chronotropic, dromotropic and bathmotropic effects with increased cardiac output and oxygen requirements;

— An increase in renin secretion;

- An increase in lipolysis (stimulates triglyceride lipase).

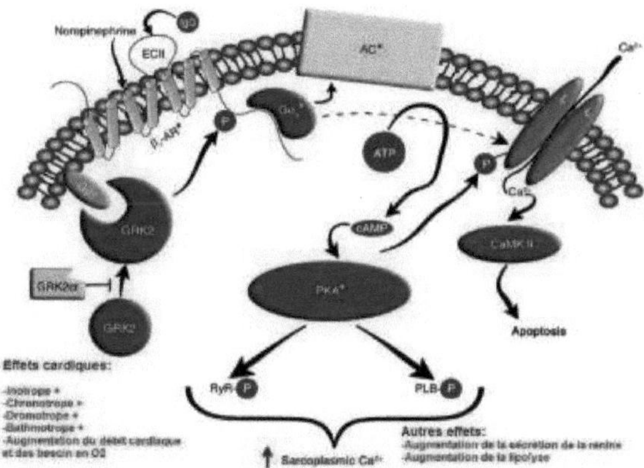

Figure 2. Stimulation of the e1-adrenergic receptor (Neil J. Freedman and Robert J. Lefkowitz, 2004).

2. Stimulation of post-synaptic β2 receptors leads to ***(Figure 3)*** :

— Relaxation of smooth fibres in the vessels, bronchi and uterus (vasodilatation, bronchodilatation and uterine relaxation);

— Metabolic effects (increased hepatic and muscular glycogenolysis) ;

— Indisputable positive inotropic and chronotropic effects, but less than those resulting from stimulation of β1 receptors;

— Reduction in kalaemia by stimulation of the Na /K^{++} pump.

3. Stimulation of pre-synaptic β2 receptors increases the release of noradrenaline ***(Figure 3)***.

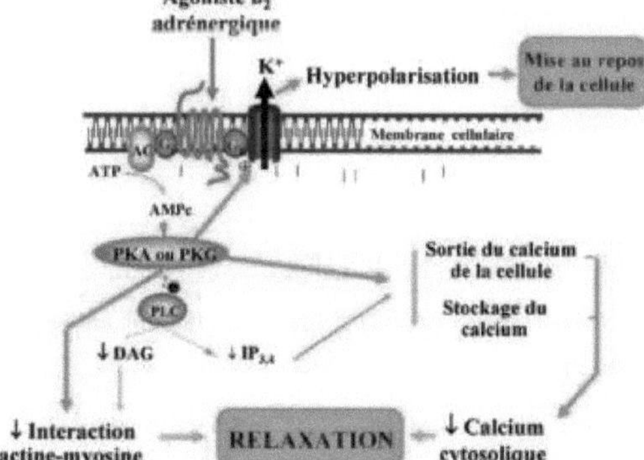

Figure 3: Stimulation of the e2-adrenergic receptor (Pierre-Olivier Girodet, 2016).

Inhibition of these receptors reduces or eliminates the effects of stimulation by endogenous catecholamines. The greater the endogenous stimulation, the greater the effect. Inhibition of the β effects may improve certain symptoms but worsen others, depending on the patient's condition.

3. Discovery history

The discovery of β-blockers stems from observations made by POWELL and SLATER in

1958 on the inhibition of the effects of *Isoprenaline* on the heart and vessels by an analogue of this substance, *Dichloro-isoprenaline* ***(figure 4)***

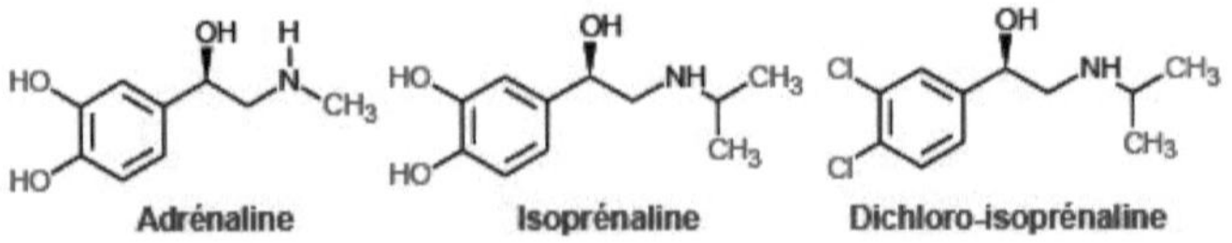

Adrénaline Isoprénaline Dichloro-isoprénaline

Figure 4: Chemical structure of adrenaline, isoprenaline and dichloroisoprenaline.

Isoprenaline was chosen as the lead compound for the synthesis of β-antagonists, as it is selective for β-receptors.

The aim was to modify *Isoprenaline* to make it an antagonist. The phenolic hydroxyls are important for agonist activity, and were replaced by other substituents such as chlorine. The resulting molecule is a partial agonist (weakened agonist activity compared with *Isoprenaline*) ***(Figure 5).***

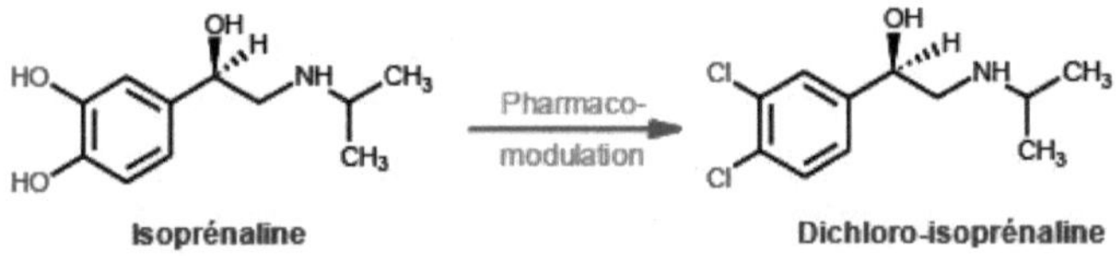

Isoprénaline Pharmaco-modulation Dichloro-isoprénaline

Figure 5. Pharmaco-modulation of Isoprenaline.

To eliminate the partial agonist activity and transform the agonist into an antagonist, a classic pharmaceutical chemistry strategy was used, namely the addition of an extra aromatic ring (more extensive hydrophobic interaction). The resulting molecule *was Pronethalol*, which was still a partial agonist, but became the first β-blocker to be used ***(Figure 6)***.

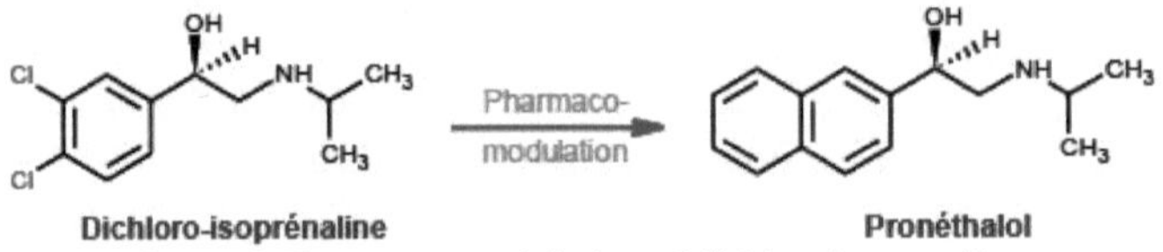

Dichloro-isoprénaline Pharmaco-modulation Pronéthalol

Figure 6. Pharmaco-modulation of dichloroisoprenaline.

Research continued and an extension of the chain linking the aromatic ring to the amine was examined, resulting in *Propranolol*, which is a pure antagonist and was 10 to 20 times more active than *Pronethalol* ***(Figure*** *7)*.

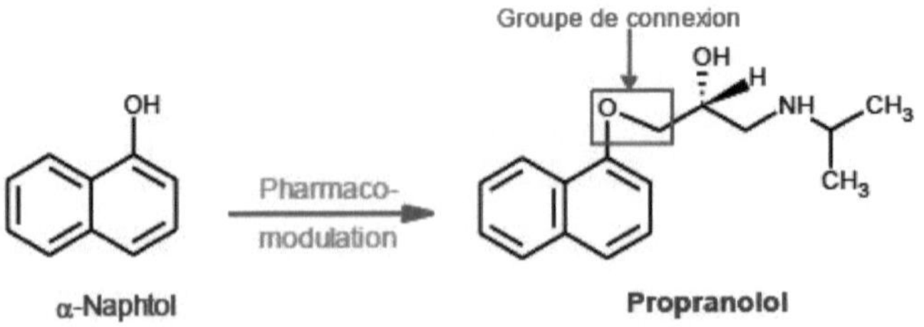

Groupe de connexion

α-Naphtol Pharmaco-modulation Propranolol

Figure 7. Production of Propranolol.

The history of β-blockers began in 1964 with BLACK's studies on *Propranolol*, followed by the introduction of this molecule into therapeutics. Initially proposed for the treatment of angina, *Propranolol* demonstrated powerful antihypertensive activity in clinical trials. As a result, β-blockers were promoted to the rank of first-line treatment for arterial hypertension.

Based on *the Propranolol* model, numerous structural analogues have been prepared and studied, and around thirty are marketed in Western countries. In addition, the evidence of an effect on intraocular pressure has led to the development a number of anti-glaucoma eye drops which now play a leading role in ophthalmic therapeutics.

4. Classification of β-blockers

4.1. Classification by chemical structure

There are two very unevenly distributed types of structure:

4.1.1. Arylethanolamines

Those most directly related to adrenaline, but the least numerous, have only a few representatives, including a compound with a mixed a- and β-blocking action, *Labetalol.* The INN of molecules belonging to this class ends with the suffix *(alol)* ***(Figure 8, Table I).***

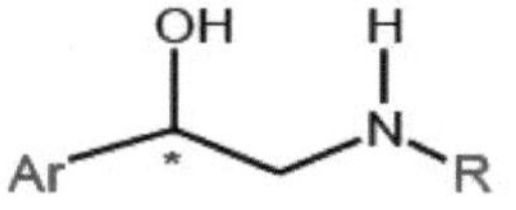

Figure 8. Chemical structure of arylethanolamine β-blockers.

Table I. Principal arylethanolamine β-blockers.

Molecule DCI	Trade name and Pharmaceutical Form	Chemical Structure and Scientific Name
Sotalol	**SOTALEX®** Comprimés à 80 mg	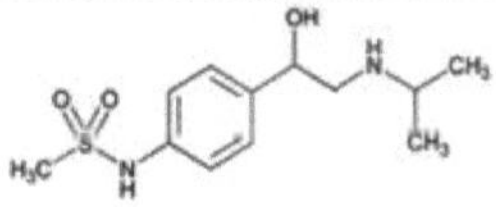 N-[4-[(1RS)-1-hydroxy-2-[(1-méthyl éthyl) amino]éthyl] phényl] Méthane sulfonamide.
Labétalol	**TRANDATE®** Comprimés à 200 mg	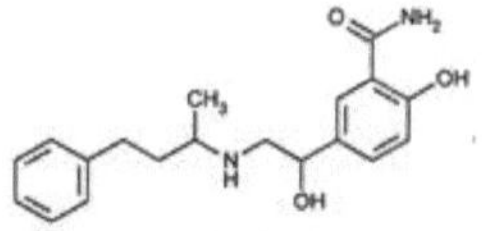 2-hydroxy-5-[1-hydroxy -2-[(1-méthyl-3-phénylpropyl) amino] éthyl] benzamide.

4.1.2. Aryloxypropanolamines

These are analogues of the previous ones, with an oxymethylene residue inserted between the aryl group and the ethanolamine chain. They have the largest number of representatives. The INN for molecules in this class ends with the suffix *(olol)* ***(Figure 9, Table II).***

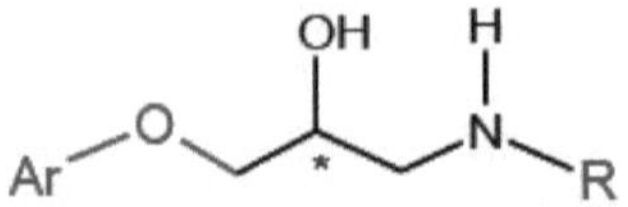

Figure 9. Chemical structure of aryloxypropanolamine β-blockers.

Figure 9. Chemical structure of aryloxypropanolamine β-blockers.

The ***Ar*** ring is either a mono- or polysubstituted benzene ring, or a simple or condensed heterocycle.

In the vast majority of cases, the ***R*** radical is an isopropyl or tert-butyl group; this structural feature is decisive for binding to β-adrenergic receptors.

Both these series contain an asymmetric carbon, but most commercial products are racemic.

Table II. Principal aryloxypropanolamine β-blockers.

Molecule DCI	Trade name and Pharmaceutical Form	Chemical Structure and Scientific Name
Acébutolol	**SECTRAL®** Comprimés à 200 mg	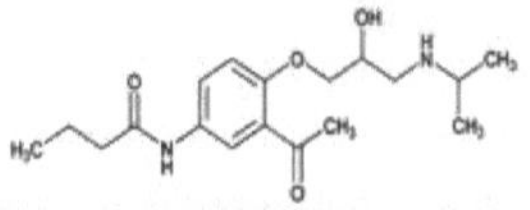 N-[3-acétyl-4-[(2RS)-2-hydroxy-3-[(1-méthyl éthyl)amino]-propoxy] phényl] butanamide.
Aténolol	**TÉNORMINE®** Comprimés à 50 mg et 100 mg	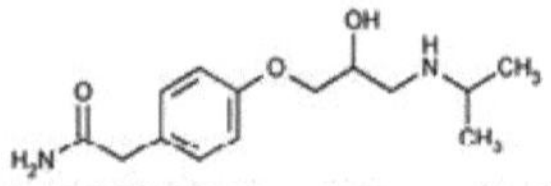 2-[4-[(2RS)-2-Hydroxy-3-[(propan-2-yl) amino] propoxy]-phényl] acétamide.

Table II. Principal aryloxypropanolamine β-blockers.

Molecule DCI	Trade name and Pharmaceutical Form	Chemical Structure and Scientific Name
Métoprolol	LOPRESSOR® Comprimés LP à 200mg	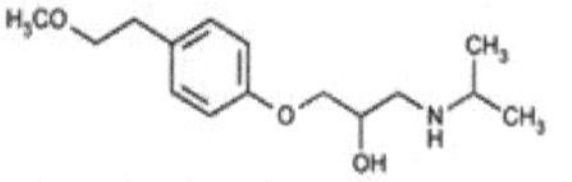 (2RS)-1-[4-(2-méthoxyéthyl)phénoxy] - 3-[(1-méthyléthyl) amino] propan-2-ol
Bétaxolol	BÉTOPTIC® Collyre à 0,5 %	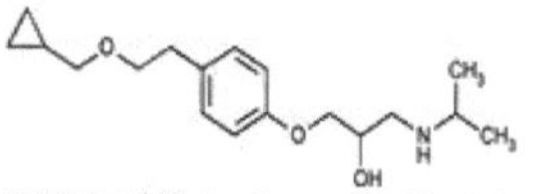 (2RS)-1-[4-[2-(cyclopropyl méthoxy)-éthyl]phénoxy]-3-[(1-méthyléthyl) amino] propan-2-ol.
Bisoprolol	DÉTENTIEL® Comprimés à 10 mg	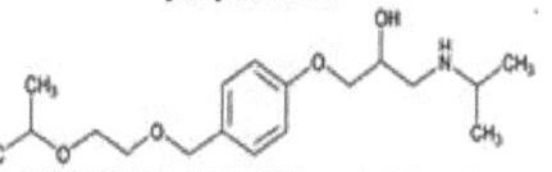 1-[4-[[2-(1-méthyléthoxy) éthoxy] méthyl] phénoxy]-3-[(1-méthyléthyl) amino]propan-2-ol.
Propranolol	AVLOCARDYL® Comprimés à 40 mg	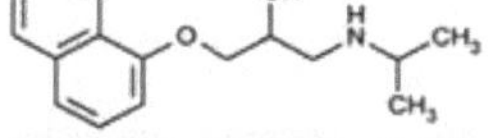 (2RS)-1-[(1-méthyléthyl) amino]-3-(naphtalèn-1-yloxy)propan-2-ol.
Timolol	TIMACOR® Comprimés à 10 mg	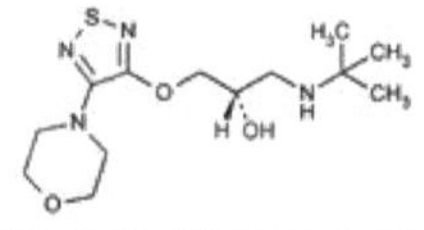 (1,1-diméthyléthyl)amino]-3-[4-(morpholin-4-yl)-1,2,5-thiadiazol-3-yl]oxy]propan-2-ol.
Cartéolol	CARTÉOL® Collyre à 2 %	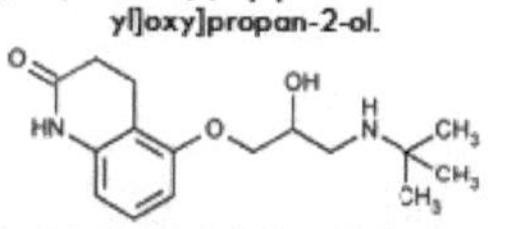 5-[3-[(1,1-diméthyléthyl)amino]-2-hydroxy-propoxy]-3,4-dihydro quinolein-2-one.

4.2. Classification according to properties pharmacological

β-blockers are classified according to three main pharmacological properties ***(Table III):***

4.2.1. Intrinsic sympathomimetic activity (ISA)

Some β-blockers used therapeutically also have a paradoxical β-stimulant or partial agonist effect. The presence of this activity could be a factor in the relative limitation of β-blocking power, mainly at rest, with no effect on the antihypertensive effect.

4.2.2. Cardio selectivity

β-blockers are classified according to their more or less selective inhibition of β1 and β2 receptors. Some β-blockers inhibit both β1 and β2 receptors, while others inhibit only β1 receptors. The latter are said to be cardio-selective, causing no adverse effects in the bronchi or peripheral vessels, but this selectivity disappears when the dose is increased.

4.2.3. Membrane stabilising effect (MSE)

It inhibits transmembrane ion exchange, resulting in a local anaesthetic action and myocardial effects similar to those of quinidine, reducing automatism, conduction and the force of myocardial contraction.

This effect can be beneficial by increasing the anti-arrhythmic effect, but it can also risk facilitating the onset of heart failure.

Table III. Classification of β-blockers according to pharmacological pharmacological properties.

Cardio-selective β-blockers			Non-cardio-selective β-blockers			
With UPS	Without UPS		With UPS		Without UPS	
With ESM	With ESM	Without ESM	With ESM	Without ESM	With ESM	Without ESM
Acebutolol		Atenolol	Alprenolol		Propranolo l	Sotalol
Metoprolol	Betaxolol	Bisoprolo l	Oxprenolol	Pindolol	Butofilolol	Timolol
		Esmolol				Nadalol

5. Access

5.1. Synthesis of aryloxypropanolamines

The general method consists of reacting epichlorohydrin (2-chloromethyloxirane) with a phenolic compound in the presence of a base. The intermediate obtained is the epoxide, which leads to the racemic amino alcohol by reaction with an appropriate amine ***(Figure 10).***

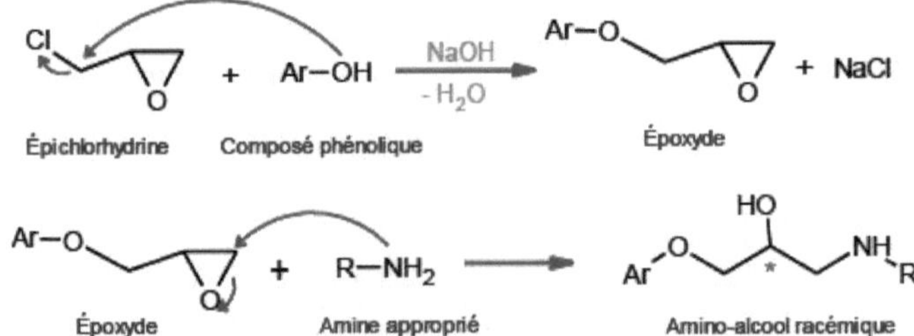

Figure 10. Synthesis of aryloxypropanolamines.

A Application to the synthesis of Propranolol

Propranolol is a β-amino alcohol belonging to the phenoxypropanolamine family.

The a-naphthol reacts with an excess of glycerol epichlorohydrin in the presence of sodium hydroxide, the intermediate obtained reacts with isopropylamine to give *Propranolol* in the form of a base.

Propranolol base is converted to a hydrochloride salt in the presence of hydrochloric acid and propan-1-ol ***(Figure 11)***.

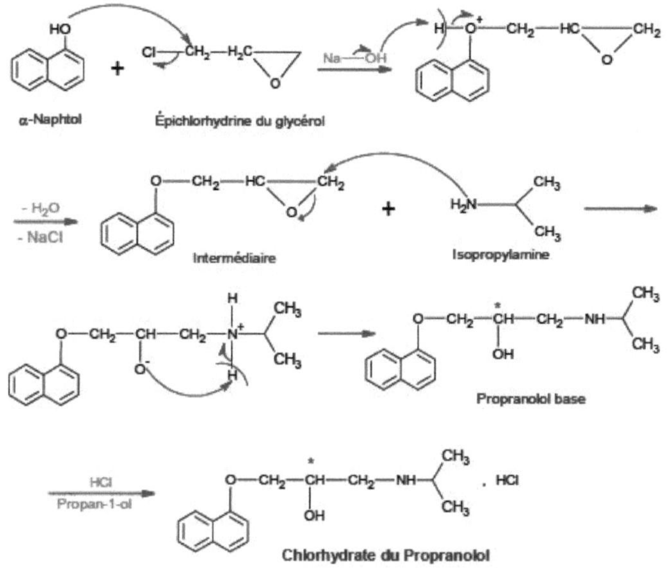

Figure 11. Synthesis of Propranolol.

5.2. **Synthesis of phenylethanolamines**

The route to this structure is similar to that of adrenaline derivatives.

A Application to the synthesis of Labetalol

5-bromoacetylsalicylamide is condensed with N-benzyl-N-(1-methyl-3-phenylpropyl)amine in the presence of butanone at reflux to produce N-(1-methyl-3-phenylpropyl)glycyl salicylamide, which is then reduced with H2/Pt in ethanol to produce *Labetalol (Figure 12)*.

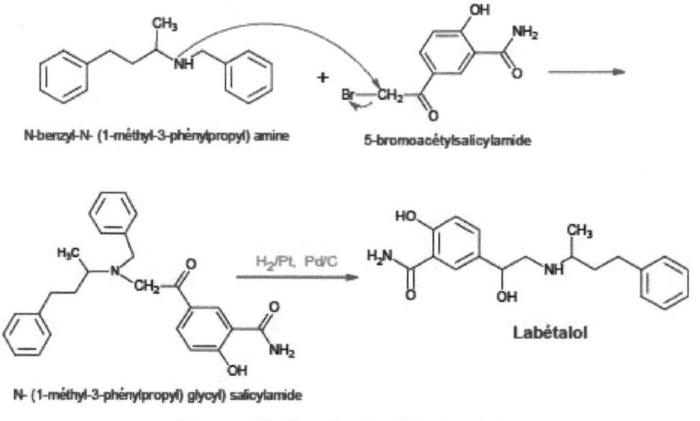

Figure 12. Synthesis of Labetalol.

6. Analytical control

6.1. Physico-chemical characteristics

β-blockers come in the form of white or slightly coloured crystalline powder.

Bases are practically insoluble in water, sparingly soluble in methanol and ethanol, and very sparingly soluble in dichloromethane. They dissolve in dilute mineral acid solutions.

Mineral or organic salts are fairly soluble in water; in the case *of Sotalol*, the hydrochloride is very soluble.

The most lipophilic *are Propranolol, Alprenolol* and *Oxprenolol.* The most hydrophilic *are Sotalol, Atenolol, Nadolol* and *Practolol.*

6.2. **Identification**

- Infrared spectrometry: comparison with SCR
- Ultraviolet spectrometry: determining absorption maxima
- Identification of the anion for compounds in salt form: hydrochloride, sulphate, maleate and tartrate.
- Thin layer chromatography on silica gel and UV revelation at 254 nm and/or by iodine vapours.
- Checking the melting point.

6.3. **Tests**

- Search for related substances by HPLC
- Determination of specific absorbance at UV maxima - Determination of specific rotatory power
- Research into heavy metals.

6.4. **Dosage**

Using non-aqueous protometry, the compounds are dissolved in glacial acetic acid and titrated with 0.1N perchloric acid. The end point of the titration is determined potentiometrically.

7. Molecular mechanism of action

The molecular mechanism of the β-adrenergic response involves cyclic AMP (cAMP), known as the second messenger, which comes from the transformation of ATP under the action of the membrane enzyme adenylate cyclase.

Activation of this enzyme is dependent on β_1-adrenergic receptors, but also on other membrane receptors sensitive to glucagon and histamine.

Adrenergic β-blockers reduce cAMP synthesis.

In myocardial cells, calcium enters through calcium channels, the opening of which is regulated by the intracellular concentration of cAMP. The reduction in the synthesis of this intracellular messenger leads to a reduction in the arrival of calcium at myocardial contractile proteins ***(Figure 13).***

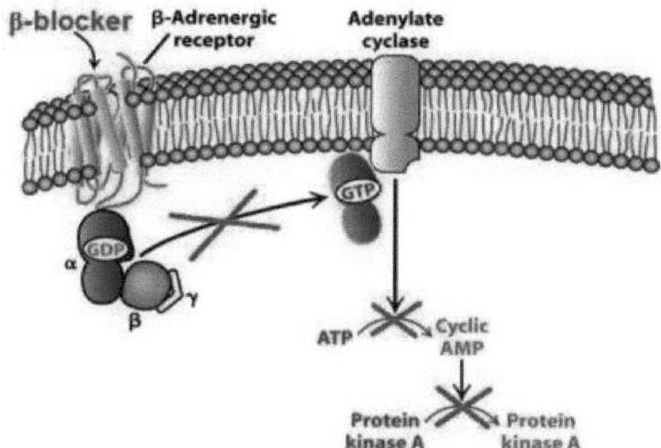

Figure 13. Molecular mechanism of action of β-blockers (W.H. Freeman, 2012).

8. Pharmacological properties

8.1. β-adrenergic inhibition

This is the main property, causing an abolition of sympathetic tone in the organs concerned; this action is reversible, and its intensity varies according to the compound used and the patient.

The distribution of the main adrenergic receptors is schematically as follows:

- Organs: Creur: β1

Vessels: α and β2

Bronchi: β2

Kidney: β1

Gil: a and β1

Digestive tract: β2

Uterus: β2

Pancreas: β2

- Cells: Metabolic effects

Glycogenolysis: β1 and β2

Lipolysis: β1 and β2

Lymphocytes: β2

We now know that the situation is not as simple as that, and that both types of β-receptor coexist in a given organ, although one is predominant.

The aim is to achieve cardio selectivity, which consists of preferential blockade of myocardial β1 receptors while respecting β2 receptors, thereby limiting adverse bronchial, vascular and metabolic effects. This relative selectivity sometimes fades when the dosage is increased.

8.2. Intrinsic sympathomimetic action

In some compounds, it co-exists to a greater or lesser extent with the predominant β-adrenergic effect. This paradoxical partial agonist action on β-adrenergic receptors enables a mixed artificial tone to be permanently maintained. To some extent, ASI may have a protective effect on atrioventricular conduction.

8.3. Stabilising effect of the membrane

Also known as "quinidine-like", it only appears at high pharmacological doses.

8.4. Effect on the renin-angiotensin system

All β-blockers reduce renin release to a greater or lesser extent.

8.5. Metabolic effects

Hepatic glycogenolysis is reduced or suppressed. Insulin secretion, which is subject to both α-adrenergic inhibitory and β-adrenergic activating tonicity, is hardly altered.

Lipolysis is inhibited, leading to an increase in plasma triglyceride levels; total cholesterol remains unchanged.

8.6. Other effects

- Decrease in intra-ocular pressure due to reduced production of aqueous humour and reduced resistance to its outflow

- Some β-blockers platelet aggregation, but this effect does not appear to be linked to β-adrenolytic action.

- Competitive α-blocker activity may coexist in certain compounds, such *as Labetalol,* which immediately reduces peripheral resistance, but its use can lead orthostatic hypotention.

9. Structure-activity relationship

9.1. Adrenergic receptor binding site

Knowledge of the binding site of adrenergic receptors is based on molecular modelling studies. From these studies, it has been shown that three transmembrane helices (TM3, TM5 and TM6) are involved in the binding site, illustrated for the β-adrenergic receptor *in **Figure 14**.*

The important residues that can bind to adrenaline or noradrenaline are :

— An aspartic acid residue (Asp-113) which interacts with the protonated nitrogen of the catecholamine via an ionic bond;

— A phenylalanine residue (Phe-290) whose aromatic ring interacts with the catechol ring via Van-der Waals interactions;

— Two serine residues (Ser-204 and Ser-207) which interact with the phenolic groups of the catecholamine via a hydrogen bond;

— An asparagine residue (Asn-293) which interacts with the alcohol function of the catecholamine.

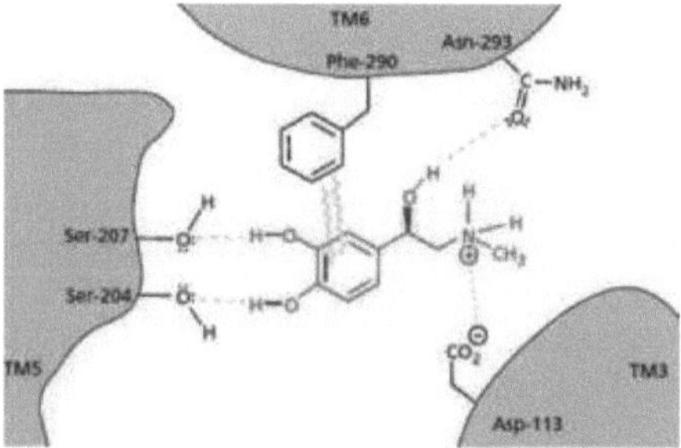

Figure 14. Adrenergic receptor binding site (Gabriel Boachie Ansah Condensed, 2018).

9.2. Important binding groups of catecholamines

Data on the above binding site interactions are provided by structure-activity relationship studies on catecholamines. They underline the importance of having ***(figure 15):***

- A secondary alcohol function that is involved in a hydrogen bond type interaction;
- An intact catechol ring with two unsubstituted phenolic OH groups, the two phenol substituents can be replaced by other groups capable interacting with the site via hydrogen bonding. The meta phenol can be replaced by groups such : CH2OH, CH2CH2OH, NH2, NHCH3, NHCOR, N(CH3)2 and NHSO2R ;
- An ionised amine.

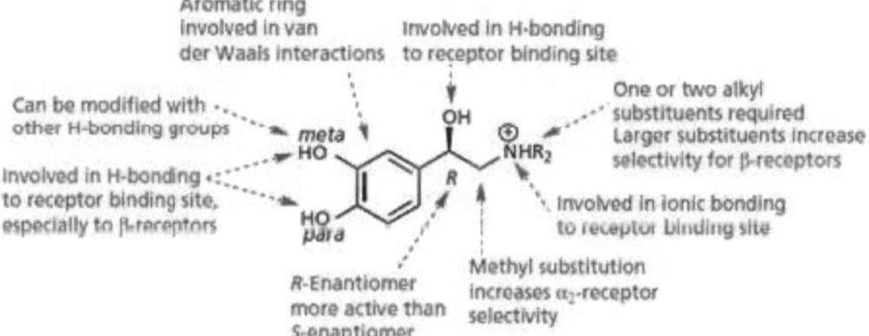

Figure 15. Important binding groups of catecholamines (Gabriel Boachie Ansah Condensed, 2018).

β-blockers are closely related structurally to catecholamines. As with catecholamines, the ß-amino alcohol linkage is a necessary condition for the manifestation of effects at adrenergic receptors. It is therefore likely that ß-blockers bind to the same ß-receptor sites as catecholamines.

The main bonds between these molecules and the receptor are at the aryl group (π interaction), the hydroxyl group (hydrogen bond) and the protonated nitrogen (ionic bond). The relative position of these three interaction poles is therefore essential to the activity of β-blockers ***(Figure 15).***

9.3. Selectivity for β-adrenergic receptors

Structure-activity relationship studies show certain characteristics that introduce selectivity between α and β receptors, with the N-alkyl substituent playing a role in this selectivity

(Figure 16).

The presence a bulky N-alkyl group, such as isopropyl or tert-butyl, is particularly selective for the β-adrenergic receptor because it has a hydrophobic pocket in which a bulky alkyl group can lodge, unlike the α-adrenergic receptor.

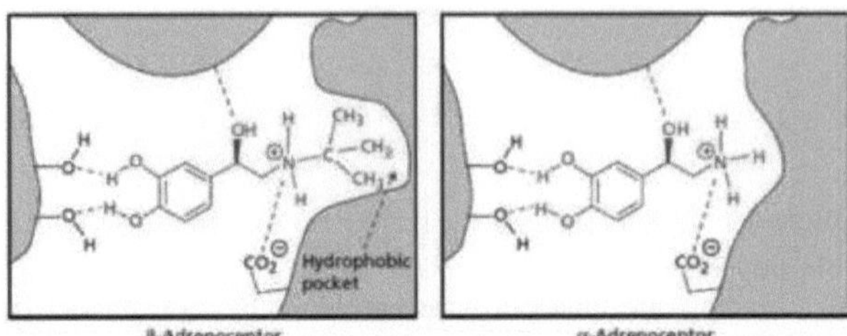

Figure 16. Comparison of α- and β-adrenergic receptor binding sites (Gabriel Boachie Ansah Condensed, 2018).

9.4. **Beta-receptor antagonism**

Most β-blockers belong to the aryloxypropanolamine chemical class:

Given that this structural feature is frequently found in β-blockers, it was assumed that the -OCH2- group is responsible for the antagonistic properties of these molecules, but this is not true, as the -OCH2- group is present in several compounds that are potent agonists, leading to the conclusion that it is the nature of the aromatic ring and its substituents that is the main determinant of antagonistic activity.

A large number of aryloxypropanolamines were synthesised and tested, and the structure-activity relationship findings were as follows ***(Figure 18):***

- Bulky branched N-alkyl substituents such as isopropyl and t-butyl are beneficial for β-antagonist activity, suggesting an interaction with a hydrophobic pocket in the binding site (identical to β-agonists);
- Variable aromatic ring systems are possible and heteroaromatic rings can be introduced, for example *Pindolol and Timolol* ***(figure 17);***

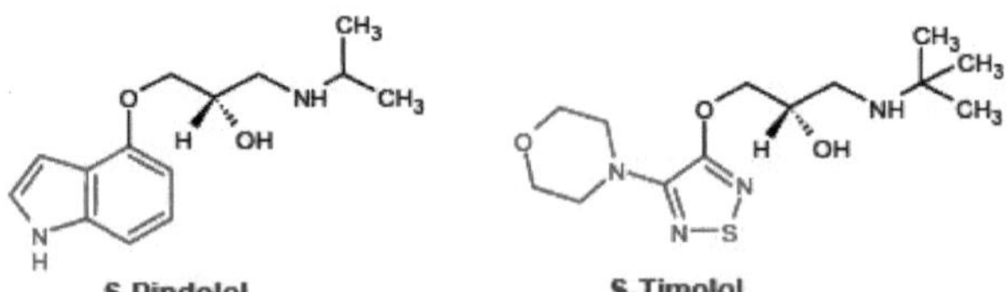

Figure 17. β-blockers with heteroaromatic rings.

- Substitution of the methylene group in the side chain increases metabolic stability but reduces activity;
- The alcohol group on the side chain is essential for the activity;
- Replacing the oxygen in the oxymethylene side chain with sulphur (S) or methyl (CH2) reduces activity, although a tissue-selective β-blocker was obtained by replacing oxygen (O)

with nitrogen (NH);

- N-alkyl substituents longer than isopropyl or t-butyl are less active, but adding an N-arylethyl group, such as [-CH(CH3)2-CH2-Ph] or [-CH2-CH2-CH2-Ph], is beneficial (extension);
- The amine must be secondary.

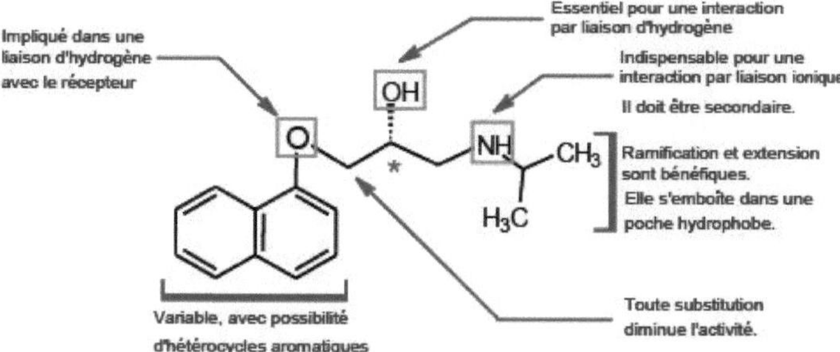

Figure 18. Structure-activity relationship of aryloxypropanolamines.

9.5. Comparison of the structures of aryloxypropanolamines and phenylethanolamines

If we consider the distance between the aromatic ring and the protonated amine function, it should be greater for aryloxypropanolamines than for phenylethanolamines, since it includes an additional non-oxymethylene chain.

However, if we examine the nature of the bonds at this precise point in the molecule by crystallography, we find a shortening of the CAr _O and O_CH2 bonds (1.36 and 1.43 A° respectively) which seems to indicate a certaindelocalisation. On the other hand, the value of the dihedral angle Γ, always close to O°, tends to prove that the flat part of the molecule extends from the aromatic ring to the methylene carbon ***(Figure 19):***

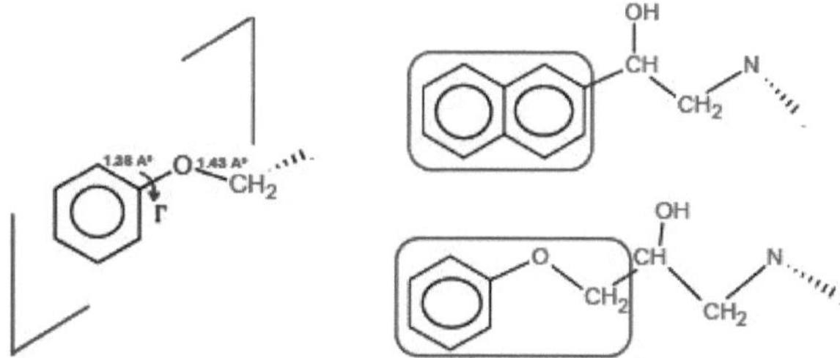

Figure 19. Comparison of the structures of aryloxypropanolamines and phenylethanolamines.

JEN and Kaiser also postulated the existence of two hydrogen bonds in the conformation of protonated aryloxypropanolamines, which would further reduce the distance between the aromatic ring and the amine function.

Calculation of the respective mean distances between the alcoholic OH, the protonated nitrogen and the point π representing the mean barycentre of the electronic cloud π,

effectively confirms the great similarity of
structure between the two families of β-blockers **(table IV)**:

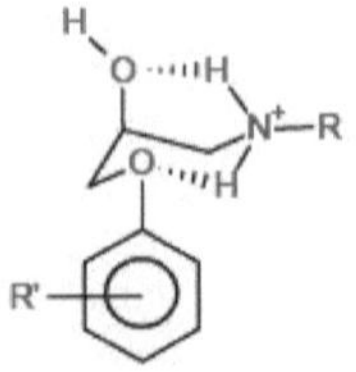

Table IV. Calculation of the distance between the aromatic ring and the amine function.

Chemical Class	O_N+	+	0_π
Phenylethanolamines	2,87 A°	6,21 A°	4,70 A°
Aryloxypropanolamines	2,90 A°	5,99 A°	4,61 A°

9.6. Stereochemistry

All β-blockers have at least one asymmetric carbon in their structure that confers optical activity to the drug. They are therefore racemic products with two isomers for each asymmetric carbon.

For maximum efficiency in binding to the receptor, the hydroxy group must occupy the same region in space as the agonists (R configuration).

Due to the insertion of an oxygen atom in the side chain of aryloxypropanolamines, the Cahn-Ingold-Prelog priority of substituents around the asymmetric carbon differs from that of agonists, and the isomer with the required spatial arrangement has the absolute S configuration ***(Figure 20)***

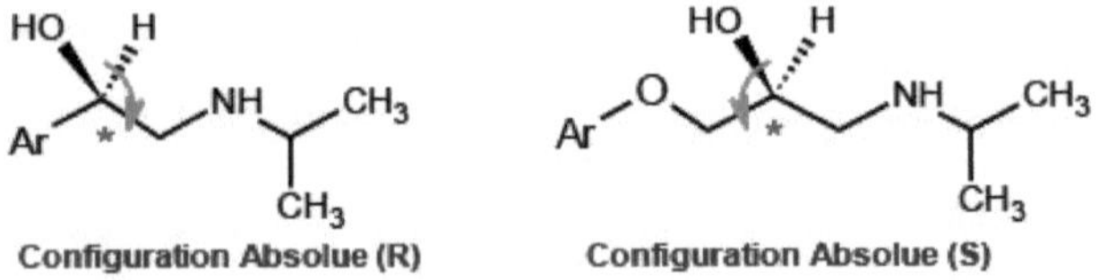

Configuration Absolue (R) Configuration Absolue (S)

Figure 20: Stereochemistry of β-adrenergic antagonists.

9.7. Blocking α-receptors

Studies of the structure-activity relationship between phenylethanolamines have shown that substitution of the nitrogen atom by a group larger than t-butyl (Aryl- α-methylalkyl group) confers affinity for ai receptors on the molecule. Consequently, compounds with a-blocking activity (*Labetalol and Carvedilol)* are mixed α/β antagonists and they were obtained by substituting the nitrogen of arylethanolamines and aryloxypropanolamines with lipophilic bulky groups.

For *Labetalol*, the arylalkyl group and the methyl group are responsible for its a1-blocking activity (as for *Dobutamine*, which is a selective α1-receptor agonist). The phenylethanolamine moiety and the bulky substituent attached to the nitrogen atom (N-arylalkyl) give it the property of a mixed α and β receptor antagonist ***(Figure 21).***

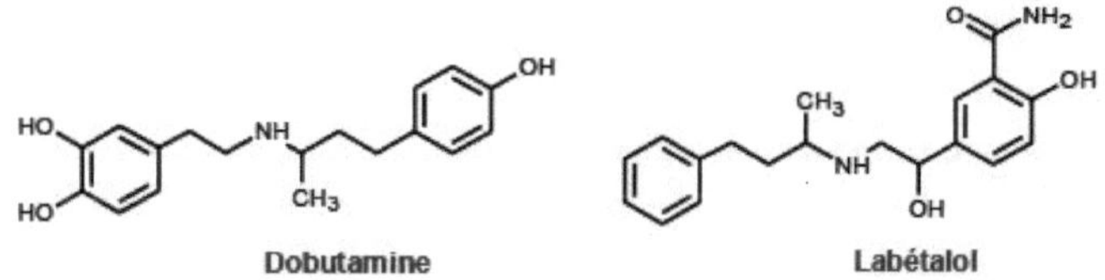

Figure 21. Chemical structures of Dobutamine and Labetalol.

In *the* case of *Carvedilol*, the aryloxypropanolamine moiety and the bulky substituent attached to the nitrogen atom give it the property antagonising both α and β receptors.

In addition to its ai- and β-blocking activity, the tricyclic carbazole moiety also gives the *Carvedilol molecule* anti-oxidant properties (***Figure 22).***

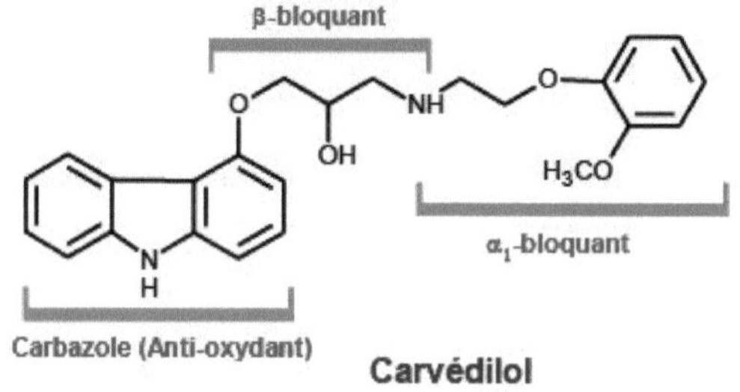

Figure 22. Chemical structure of Carvedilol.

10. Indications

10.1. Treatment of hypertension

The antihypertensive action results from the following effects:

Action on the heart by reducing cardiac output,

- Action on the kidneys by reducing the release of renin;

- Inhibitory effects on the stimulation of pre-synaptic e2-adrenergic receptors by adrenaline.

10.2. Prophylactic treatment of angina attacks

- β-blockers are the reference treatment for stress angina and the chronic preventive treatment for post-myocardial infarction events.

- Their effectiveness is based on their negative inotropic and chronotropic effects, which reduce cardiac activity and therefore myocardial oxygen requirements.

10.3. Treatment of arrhythmias

- β-blockers have an effect on all catecholinergic rhythm disorders ( ). They correspond to Group II of the Vaughan-Williams classification of anti-arrhythmics (except Sotalol).

- The anti-arrhythmic effect is explained by a reduction in sinus automatism and nodal conductivity.

10.4. Treatment of heart failure

For a long time, β-blockers were considered to be contraindicated heart failure because they reduced cardiac output and myocardial contractility. However, the hypothesis of an improvement in symptoms has been tested in several clinical trials, and four β-blockers (*Carvedilol, Bisoprolol, Metoprolol LP and Nebivolol*) have demonstrated their efficacy and have marketing authorisation for this indication.

10.5. **Other non-cardiovascular indications**

10.6. Treatment of glaucoma (Carteolol and Betaxolol): the chance discovery of a drop in ocular pressure in glaucoma patients with arterial hypertension treated with β-blockers led to the use of these drugs in the long-term treatment of chronic glaucoma.

10.7. Propranolol and Metoprolol are used to reduce the number and intensity of migraine attacks, due to their vasoconstrictive effect.

11. Contraindications

- Asthma: β-blockers are contraindicated in patients with asthma or a history of asthma, in whom they may induce or aggravate asthma.
- Significant sinus bradycardia (less than 45 beats per min)
- Severe chronic obstructive pulmonary disease
- Second-degree atrioventricular block
- Severe peripheral arterial disease
- Patients with Raynaud's syndrome.

12. Undesirable effects

— Possible aggravation of a rhythm disorder by excessive bradycardia

— Sinus bradycardia and reduced conduction may induce or aggravate sino-atrial blocks or atrioventricular blocks.

— The haemodynamic consequences of allergic shock are more significant insofar as sympathetic cardiac inotropic stimulation is blocked, preventing blood pressure from being maintained.

— The imbalance in favour of the alpha-vasoconstrictor effect can lead to Raynaud's syndromes.

— Sleep disorders and depression have also been reported with β-blockers, especially if they have a passage into the CNS (fat-soluble β-blockers).

— Aggravation of psoriasis lesions (by reducing the production of cAMP in the skin)

— Symptoms of hypoglycaemia in treated diabetics (tachycardia and tremors) are reduced, and therefore less perceptible, which is why they should be treated with caution.

— Metabolic disorders.

13. Conclusion and outlook

What β-blockers have in common is that they block βι-adrenergic receptors, but they have different pharmacological properties. Numerous studies have compared them to determine which would be the best choice depending on the pathology to be treated and the characteristics of the patients. The following conclusions can be drawn:

In terms of efficacy, the different β-blockers are very similar. It is the βι-blocking property that is responsible for all the therapeutic effects, particularly antihypertensive and anti-ischaemic effects.

In terms of tolerability, there may be an advantage to using a selective ß1-blocker (one that does not block β2 receptors):

— In patients with asthma, to avoid suppression of the bronchodilator effect of β2 stimulation;

— In diabetics, to reduce the suppression of hypoglycaemic symptoms associated with reactive sympathetic stimulation (tachycardia, palpitations, anxiety and tremors);

— In patients with peripheral arterial disease, to preserve arteriolar vasodilation dependent on stimulation of e2-adrenergic receptors;

- In patients with elevated blood cholesterol and triglycerides, to preserve the action of lipoprotein lipase.

In practice, the differences between selective and non-selective β-blockers are not 'clinically' very significant, as selectivity is only relative and decreases with increasing doses.

The partial β1 agonist effect is of no interest here, since it would limit the β1 blocking effect that we are looking for.

A partial β2 agonist effect would be interesting for lipid metabolism.

Today, β-blockers seem to reached a high level of development, and it is likely that no major breakthrough will be expected in the next few years, at least in the series that have traditionally been explored. Nevertheless, there is still room for improvement, particularly in terms of cardioselectivity.

14. References

1. TRONCHE P et COUQUELET J. Les Bêta-bloquants. **In**: BRION JD, BUXERAUD J, CASTEL J et al. *Médicaments du Système Cardio- Vasculaire*, Paris: Tec & Doc, 1992, p. 105-139. (Traité de Chimie Thérapeutique, Volume 3).
2. WATSON, David G. Drugs Affecting The Adrenergic System. **In**: *Pharmaceutical Chemistry* **[Online]**. 1st ed. United Kingdom: Churchill Livingstone Elsevier, 2011, p. 199-214. Available from: < https://www.elsevier.com/books/pharmaceutical-chemistry/watson/ 978-0-443-07233-8> (Accessed 20/12/2019).
3. KIRKIACHARIAN, Serge. Medicines for the Cardiovascular System. **In**: *Guide de Chimie Médicinale et Médicaments*, Paris: Tec & Doc, 2010, p. 249-264.
4. KIRKIACHARIAN, Serge and PIERI, François. Medicines for the Autonomic Nervous System. **In**: *Pharmacologie et Thérapeutique.* 2th ed. Paris: Ellipses, 1992, p. 140-144.
5. TAOUFIK, Jamal. Médicaments du Système Nerveux Autonome. **In**: *Précis de Chimie Thérapeutique*, Rabat: MEDIKA, 2007, p. 203-205.
6. LECHAT, Philippe. *Pharmacologie.* **[On-line].** Paris: Université Pierre et Marie Curie, Service de pharmacologie, Niveau DCEM1, 2006, 349 p. Available at: < http://www.chups.jussieu.fr/polys/pharmaco /poly/ Pharmaco .pdf> (Accessed 25/12/2019).
7. GORRE, Frauke and VANDEKERCKHOVE, Hans. Beta-blockers: focus on mechanism of action Which beta-blocker, when and why? *Acta Cardiologica* **[Online]**. 2010; 65(5): 565-570. Available at:< https://www.researchgate.net/p ublication/49652938Betablockerfocusonmechanismofaction Whichbeta-blockerwhenandwhy> (Accessed 25/12/2019).
8. RESHMI, Sameeth. *Beta blockers.* **[Online]**. 2016, 68 p. Available at:< https://fr.slideshare.net/DrReshmiSameeth/beta-blockers- > 57403519(Accessed on 25/12/2019).
9. CIZMARIRKOVA Ruzena, HABALA Ladislav, VALENTOVA Jindra and MARKULIAK Mario. Survey of pharmacological activity and pharmacokinetics of selected adrenergic blockers in regard to their stereochemistry. *Applied Sciences* **[Online]**. 2019; 9(625): 1-29. Available from:< https://scholar.google.com/scholar?Surveyof+Pharmacological+Activity+and+Pharmacokinetics+of+Selected+%0CAdrener

gic+Blockers+in+Regard+to+Their+Stereochemistry&hl= en&assdt &asvis=1&oi=scholart=0 > (Accessed 27/12/2019).

10. European Directorate for the Quality of Medicines and Healthcare. Propranolol hydrochloride monograph. **In**: *European Pharmacopoeia.* 9th ed. France: EDQM, 2018, p. 3675-3676.

11. European Directorate for the Quality of Medicines and Healthcare. Labetalol hydrochloride monograph. **In**: *European Pharmacopoeia.* 9th ed. France: EDQM, 2018, p. 3065-3067.

Chapter 3

Central anti-hypertensives

1. Introduction

Apart from a few special cases, centrally-acting antihypertensives are indicated as third- or fourth-line treatments for essential hypertension and are used in combination with other antihypertensives. They are presynaptic alpha-2 agonists acting on the bulbar cardiomodulatory centres and all have a more or less marked central sympatholytic effect.

2. Pathophysiological background

A "catecholamine" is defined by a catechol ring, which is a benzene aromatic ring with two adjacent hydroxyl groups and a short hydrocarbon chain ending in an amine group **(Figure 1).**

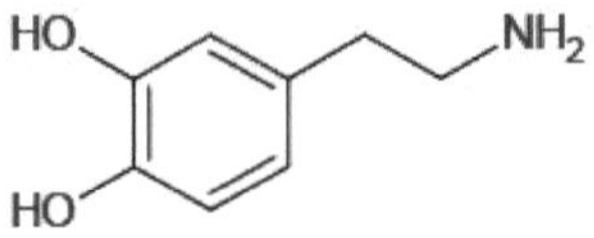

HO, HO, NH_2

Figure 1: Catecholamine core.

Catecholamines are :

- Norepinephrine or noradrenaline is the neurotransmitter of sympathetic post-ganglionic fibres and certain neurons of the central nervous system;
- Epinephrine or adrenaline is the main hormone secreted into the systemic circulation by the adrenal medulla;
- Dopamine is the natriuretic catecholamine, acting locally in the kidneys but also centrally as a neurotransmitter.

2.1. Adrenergic receptors

The physiological and metabolic effects of catecholamines are determined by specific receptors, called adrenergic receptors, inserted into the membrane of the effector cells. In 1945, AHLQUIST was the first to propose the existence of two types of adrenergic receptor, α and β, to explain the different physiological effects mediated by adrenaline and noradrenaline.

AHLQUIST determined the effects attributable to α or β-adrenergic receptors according to an order of potency of the following agonists: Adrenaline> Noradrenaline> Isoprenaline defining α-adrenergic receptors, while Isoprenaline > Adrenaline >> Norepinephrine for β-adrenergic receptors.

As a result, adrenaline stimulates both types of adrenergic receptor, whereas noradrenaline preferentially stimulates α-adrenergic receptors.

2.3. Subtypes of a-adrenergic receptors

Pharmacological evidence has also provided clues to the existence of different types of α-adrenergic receptors:

— The α-adrenergic receptors al ;
— a2-adrenergic receptors.

In the sympathetic system, α1 adrenergic receptors are predominantly post-synaptic, whereas a2 receptors are predominantly pre-synaptic **(Figure 2).**

In the central nervous system, a2 receptors predominate.

These different locations explain why a substance that interacts with a-adrenergic receptors will have different effects depending on which receptors it stimulates or blocks.

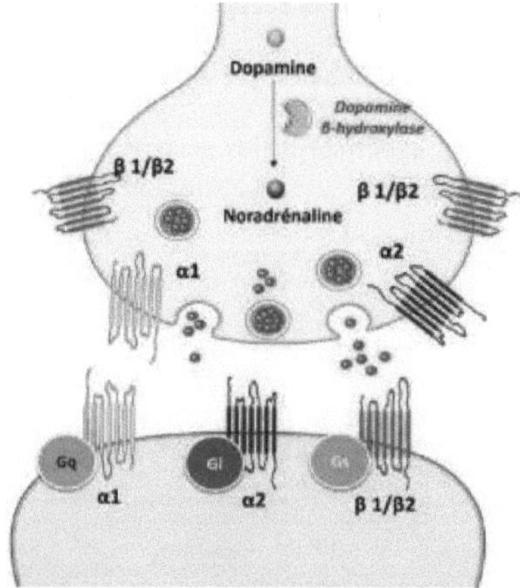

Figure 2: Synaptic distribution of noradrenergic receptors (R BORDET, 2019).

2.4. Effects of receptor stimulation

2.4.1. Effects of stimulating α1 peripherals

Contraction of smooth fibres :

— Vascular fibres (increased arterial pressure and peripheral resistance) ;

— Trigone vesica (promotes urination) ;

— Bladder neck and urethra (promotes bladder continence and prevents retrograde ejaculation);

— Intestine: contraction of sphincter muscles (evacuation);

— Iris dilator muscle (mydriasis) ;

— Smooth pilomotor muscle (ruffles the hair) ;

- Creur: increases the strength of contractions (very slight effect in humans) Hepatic glycogenolysis (increase in blood sugar).

2.4.2. Effects of stimulating α2 peripherals

- Contraction of certain vascular smooth fibres (non-innervated fibres)

- Adipocytes: inhibition of lipolysis

- Relaxation of intestinal smooth muscle (by reducing acetylcholine release: pre-synaptic alpha-adrenergic action)

- Reduces water and salt secretion (used in the treatment of certain types of diarrhoea such as cholera).

- Stimulation of platelet aggregation
- Decreased renin secretion
- Decreased release of noradrenaline (pre-synaptic effect)
- Decreased insulin secretion.

2.4.3. Effects of stimulation of central α2 receptors

- Sedation
- Reduction in sympathetic tone (drop in blood pressure) arterial)
- Reduced secretion from certain exocrine glands such as the salivary glands (leading to dry mouth) **(Figure 3).**

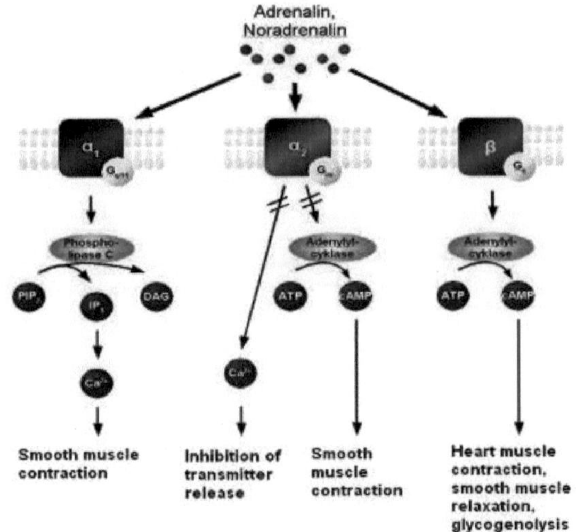

Figure 3: Effects of adrenergic receptor stimulation (J DEGUIL, 2019).

3. Central anti-hypertensives

3.1. General

Central anti-hypertensives are a2-adrenergic agonists with a weak vasoconstrictor effect in the periphery by stimulating post-synaptic α2 receptors, but they reduce the release of catecholamines by their presynaptic effects, which may compensate for the first effect.

The a2-adrenergics easily cross the blood-brain barrier and reduce the release of catecholamines in the blood pressure regulation centres, thereby reducing sympathetic tone and the release of catecholamines in the periphery. They are known as central hypotensives or sympatholytics; the reference drug in this class *is a-methyldopa (ALDOMET®)* **(Table I).**

Table I. Main central antihypertensive agents.

Molecule DCI	Trade name and Pharmaceutical Form	Chemical Structure and Scientific Name
α-Méthyldopa	**ALDOMET®** Comprimés à 250 mg	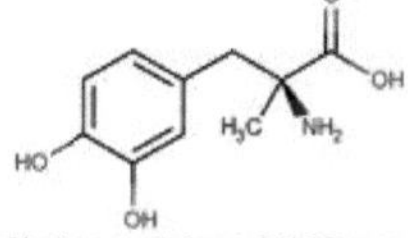 3-Hydroxy-alpha-méthyl-L-tyrosine.
Clonidine	**CATAPRESSAN®** Comprimés à 0,5 mg. Injectable 0,15 mg/mL	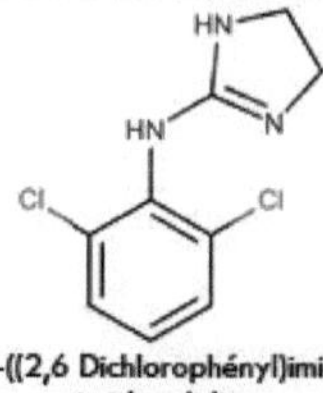 2-((2,6 Dichlorophényl)imino) imidazolidine.

Table I. Main central anti-hypertensives (Continued).

Molecule DCI	Trade name and Pharmaceutical Form	Chemical Structure and Scientific Name
Rilménidine	**HYPERIUM®** Comprimés à 1 mg	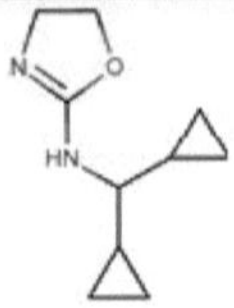 N-(dicyclopropylméthyl)-4,5-dihydro-1,3-oxazol-2-amine.
Moxonidine	**PHYSIOTENS®** Comprimés à 0,4 mg	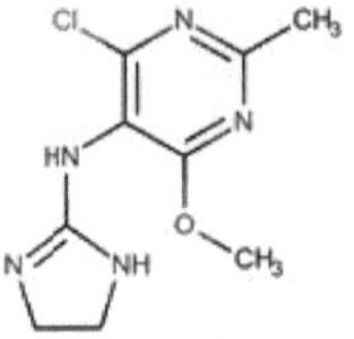 4-Chloro-N-(4,5-dihydro-1H-imidazol-2-yl)- 6-méthoxy-2-méthylpyrimidin-5-amine.
Apraclonidine Para-amino-Clonidine	**IOPIDINE®** Collyre à 0,5 %	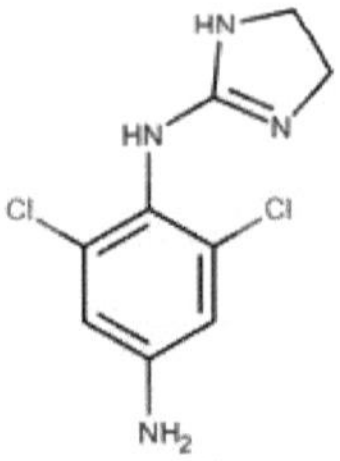 2-[(4-amino-2,6 dichlorophényl) imino]imidazolidine.

3.2. Study of the lead partner

α-Methyldopa: ALDOMET® (in French)

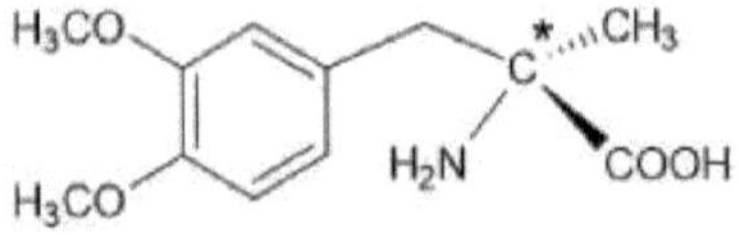

Figure 4: Chemical structure of a-methyldopa.

3.2.1. Chemical synthesis

A-methyldopa is prepared by a chloromethylation reaction of dimethoxybenzene; this reaction is carried out in three steps, the first of which is a nucleophilic addition of hydrochloric acid to acetone followed by a second addition of zinc chloride to form an oxonium intermediate which will be attacked by dimethoxybenzene to form 4-(chloromethyl)-1,2-dimethoxybenzene with the release of zinc chloride hydroxide.

The second reaction is a cyanidation with potassium cyanide followed by a Claisen condensation with ethyl methanoate in the presence of sodium ethanolate to give oxobutanoic acid.

Decarboxylation of the product formed is followed by a Bucherer reaction to form a compound with a hydontoYne ring.

Hydrolysis and methylation of this intermediate will give a racemic mixture *of a-methyldopa* which must be resolved to give the S enantiomer **(Figure 5).**

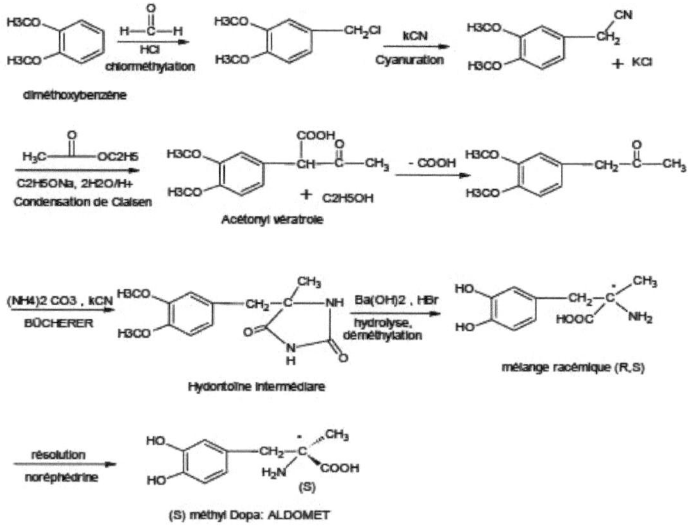

Figure 5. Chemical synthesis of l'α-methyldopa.

3.2.2. Analytical control

1. Physico-chemical properties

A-methyldopa is a fine white to yellowish-white powder, easily soluble in water, soluble in DMSO (75 mM) and dilute hydrochloric acid.

2. Identification

- Infrared spectrophotometry compared with *the* spectrum of *a-methyldopa SCR.*
- Melting point approx. 300°C.

3. Test

- Assay of related substances by liquid chromatography.
- Rotatory power test.
- Loss on drying and sulphuric ash test.

4. Dosage

Titration by potentiometry with 0.1 M sodium hydroxide.

1.3. Structure-activity relationship

A primary or secondary aliphatic amine separated by two carbons from a substituted benzene ring is essential for high agonist activity.

The hydroxyl-substituted carbon must be in the R configuration for maximum direct activity.

1.3.1. Substitution of the R1 radical

When the size of the R1 radical is increased, alpha receptor activity decreases and beta receptor activity increases.

The large lipophilic groups make it possible obtain compounds with alpha blocking activity.

The arylalkyl group can provide beta selectivity, increased cellular penetration and increased lipophilicity for a longer duration of action.

1.3.2. Substitution of the R2 radical

The ethyl group may eliminate the alpha activity of the drug.

The additional methyl group makes the drug more selective for alpha2 activity.

1.3.3. The R3 radical of the aromatic ring

The natural 3',4'-dihydroxy-substituted benzene ring of norepinephrine provides excellent α- and β-receptor activity. However, these catechol-containing compounds have low oral activity, as they are rapidly metabolised by COMT.

The 3', 5'-dihydroxy compounds are orally active.

At least one of the groups must be able to form hydrogen bonds.

If R3 is only a 3'-OH or a 3'-sulfonamide, activity is reduced at α sites but almost eliminated at β sites, resulting in selective α-agonists **(Figure 6).**

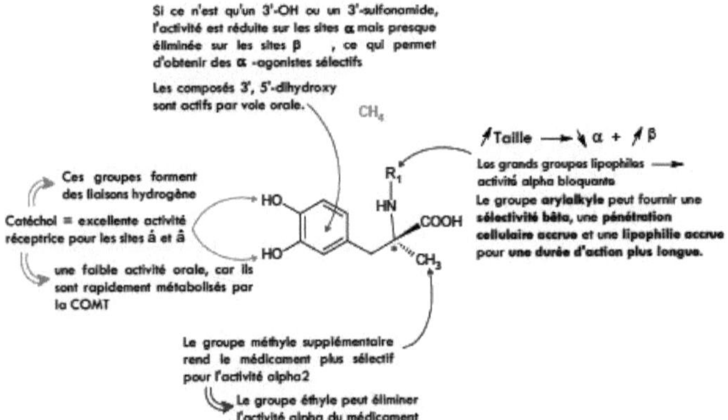

Figure 6. Structure-activity relationship of central anti-hypertensives.

1.4. Mechanism of action

Central anti-hypertensives act preferentially on a2-adrenergic receptors, and are likely to increase a depressive state or make a latent depressive state appear. In contrast, antagonists of central presynaptic α2-receptors have an antidepressant effect. *Moxonidine* should not be used in patients with heart failure.

Abrupt discontinuation of α2 agonists, particularly *Clonidine*, may be followed by a rebound in arterial hypertension, tachycardia, sweating and agitation. Re-administration of *Clonidine* eliminates the previous symptoms, which are similar to those seen when morphine is stopped. *Clonidine* can be used to reduce the intensity of the symptoms observed during morphine withdrawal.

1.5. Indications

Central antihypertensives directly reduce the effect of the orthosympathetic system, and indirectly increase that of the parasympathetic system, sensitising the bulbar centres to the inhibition of blood pressure by the baroreceptor reflex. They also have a negative inotropic and chronotropic effect, which is also clinically useful, and is more marked for *Clonidine* than *for Methyldopa.*

Methyldopa is used in the clinical treatment of the following disorders:

- Hypertension ;
- Gestational hypertension (or pregnancy-induced hypertension) and pre-eclampsia.

The main indication for *clonidine* is hypertensive emergencies.

However, *clonidine* is best known and used in anaesthesia and intensive care for its sedative and analgesic properties. It can be used per os as a premedication, intravenously and perimedullary.

1.6. Undesirable effects

Drowsiness, dry mouth and risk of hypotension are present with all centrally-acting antihypertensives. They tend to disappear over time, even after increasing the dose following the initial drug escape. If they persist, treatment may have to be discontinued.

Patients may experience depression, anxiety and asthenia. Decreased libido and erectile difficulties are relatively common.

Methyldopa has marked anti-dopaminergic properties. It may therefore cause extra-pyramidal signs (e.g. Parkinson's syndrome, dystonia) and galactorrhoea secondary to hyperprolactinaemia. There is a risk of angina, oedema, rare but serious digestive disorders and liver damage, especially during the first three months of treatment. It is associated with haemolytic anaemia.

1.7. Contraindications

- Clonidine: cardiac conduction disorders with bradycardia.
- Methyldopa: depression; acute liver diseaseê (RCP).
- Moxonidine: cardiac conduction disorders with bradycardia, severe heart failure.

4. Conclusion

Central antihypertensive agents are distinguished by their unique mechanism of action, which focuses on the central regulation of blood pressure. These agents act on the central nervous system to modulate the release of catecholamines, thereby inducing a hypotensive response.

They are presynaptic alpha-2 agonists acting on the bulbar cardiomodulatory centres and all have a more or less marked central sympatholytic effect. With no major peripheral action, they preserve the postural adaptation of blood pressure and the baroreflex.

Methyldopa remains one of the anti-hypertensives of choice, thanks to its long track record in pregnant women.

The action of central anti-hypertensives can be significant at the time of peak plasma levels, with risk of arterial hypotension, and diminishes during the course of treatment. There is a risk of rebound in the of abrupt withdrawal or missed doses. Their effects are dose-dependent, and treatment should be started at a low dose. They all cause drowsiness, depression and anhedonia, and sometimes other more serious central effects.

5. References

1. LARONZE J.Y. Les antihypertenseurs centraux. **In**: BRION JD, BUXERAUD J, CASTEL J et al. *Médicaments du Système Cardio- Vasculaire*, Paris: Tec & Doc, 1992, p. 247-260. (Traité de Chimie Thérapeutique, Volume 3).
2. KIRKIACHARIAN, Serge. Medicines for the Cardiovascular System. **In**: *Guide de Chimie Médicinale et Médicaments*, Paris: Tec & Doc, 2010, p. 249-264.
3. KIRKIACHARIAN, Serge and PIERI, François. Medicines for the Autonomic Nervous System. **In**: *Pharmacologie et Thérapeutique.* 2th ed. Paris: Ellipses, 1992, p. 140-144.
4. Collège National de Pharmacologie Médicale. Central antihypertensives. **[On line].** Bordeaux : 2019, 20 p. Available on : <https://pharmacomedicale.org/medicaments/parspecialites/item /anti-hypertensives-d-action-centrale> (Consulted on 01 /06/2024).
5. Lemke TL, Williams DA. Foye's Principles of Medicinal Chemistry. Lippincott Williams & Wilkins; 2008. 1406 p.
6. European Directorate for the Quality of Medicines and Healthcare. Methyldopa Product Monograph. **In**: *European Pharmacopoeia.* 9th ed. France: EDQM, 2018, p. 3675-3676.
7.

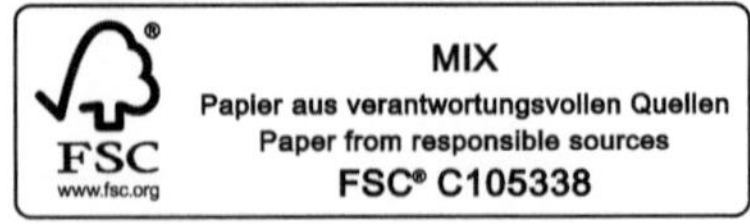

Printed by Books on Demand GmbH, Norderstedt / Germany